BRINGING YOUR
PRACTICE INTO
FOCUS

BRINGING YOUR PRACTICE INTO
FOCUS

JOHN A. WILDE, DDS

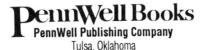
PennWell Books
PennWell Publishing Company
Tulsa, Oklahoma

Copyright © 1994 by
PennWell Publishing Company
1421 South Sheridan/P.O. Box 1260
Tulsa, Oklahoma 74101

Wilde, John A.
    Bringing your practice into focus/John A. Wilde.
        p.   cm.
    Includes index.
    ISBN 0-87814-410-2
    1. Dentistry—Practice. 2. Dentists—Finance, Personal.
I. Title.
    [DNLM: 1. Practice Management, Dental. WU 77 w6716 1993]
RK57.5.W55 1993
617.6'0068—dc20
DNLM/DLC
for Library of Congress   93-41077
                                                                          CIP

Printed in the United States of America

    2 3 4 5 98 97 96 95 94

CONTENTS

———— SECTION THREE: ————
Investment Strategies for Financial Success • 187

DEDICATION

My youngest brother, Dr. Jerry Wilde, has been an inspiration to me as well as to everyone his life has touched. If I ever felt tired or reluctant to work, just thinking of Jerry filled me with energy and love. In addition to his role as my personal motivator, Jerry has often filled the role of Muse. Many of the insights he has shared with me over the years have both improved and blessed this book with their presence. May God bless him.

Dr. Duane A. Schmidt gave me the incentive and encouragement to begin writing and started me on a marvelous adventure. Schmidty is a true giant among men, and a constant source of energy and joy to those around him. He is truly "Sooper!"

Dental Economics gave me my first chance to be published nationally and really got me hooked on writing. Of the many wonderful people on their staff I've come to know and enjoy, Penny Elliot Anderson and Dick Hale have done the most to encourage and enhance my efforts. I offer them my deepest thanks and look forward to many more years of their friendship.

My book editor, Sue Rhodes Sesso, at PennWell is the person most responsible for this book arriving in print. I'd like to thank her for all the patience and help given to one who studied science instead of English. I'm sure that choice of majors was constantly apparent in my writing.

My loyal and supportive staff at our office "laboratory" have enabled me to assimilate most of the feeble bits of wisdom I've tried to pass on here. Thanks for all their caring and patience goes to Betsy Carter, Dawn Doore, Kathleen Leitru, Carol May, Linda Schrader, Kathy Scott, Joann Wilde, Vicky Yordy, and my ever-loyal associate, Dr. Lowell Long. I couldn't have done it without you.

I'd like to give special thanks to my family for their support and encouragement. To my mom and dad, Jeanne and Mit Wilde, for instilling in me the values that 40 years later make up so much of this book's content. To my wife and children for allowing me the many hours of solitude the lonely work of writing requires. (It's been said that I'm an easy guy to be without, but I'm still grateful.) My deepest love and thanks to my wife Joann and children John, Heather, Megan, and Rachel. When I'm sad, they are my inspiration. When I thank God for all He has blessed me with, they are first on my list. They are my loves and my life.

INTRODUCTION

I hope this book will be accepted as a gift. I'd like to offer it as such. Most dentists I've known don't receive the appreciation, financial rewards, or the joy and peace that should accompany such difficult labor done daily to the best of their abilities. My desire is that by sharing some of the lessons I've learned, each of you will be able to immediately improve the quality of your life and start to enjoy more fully the fruits I feel you have already earned by your great efforts.

This is a book about rewards and joy. Make no mistake about that. It's also a book about misfortune and pain. Taken together, these are the things we call "life." I'd like you to join me on a journey through my life, both personally and professionally. To not show you both sides of my existence would, to me, be less than honest. I will demonstrate how I have been able to achieve complete financial freedom and how *you can do the same.* I also hope to show you that all the riches in the world, by themselves, are worthless. Financial well-being must be accompanied by wisdom and understanding if it is to have a positive impact on your life.

This is not to say I despise wealth. Nothing could be farther from the truth. It is rather to say that I understand money. I clearly comprehend what wealth can do. I also know what it can not accomplish. I hope, through this book, to help you clarify your own values and to aid your understanding of what money really is. Then, should you choose to attain wealth and wish to use dentistry as a means to that end, I'll show you how to achieve the riches you desire. But more than showing you how to simply attain riches, I wish to demonstrate how wealth, used in context with the proper philosophy, can bring you joy. Isn't that what we are all really seeking?

Section

1

DEVELOPMENT OF A PHILOSOPHY OF SUCCESS

CHAPTER 1

WHO IS
THIS GUY?

The most expeditious way for me to answer the above query is to state that I am a fellow "spit-soaked" dentist (20-plus years in the soaking, though now completely protected by gloves). But more meaningful than that: I'm a guy who finds performing quality dentistry very hard work. I have had the pleasant experience of achieving great financial success in my profession. I'm very grateful for that. I plan to tell you how that success came to be and how we are currently able to generate a *net of $2,000 per day* in our little country practice. Allow me to clearly state here and now that I am a *net* guy. Production, collection, overhead percentages, new patient flow: all are important milestones on the journey to financial success in dentistry. But in this book we'll concern ourselves with the real bottom line, or what is left when all the bills are paid: *net*. If you desire a financial success similar to what we have achieved, this book can serve as a blueprint for you to follow.

If I write this book well, each of you will develop a completely different blueprint. This uniqueness is essential if this book is to achieve its goal. My purpose in writing was not so you could see how I had achieved financial independence and freedom, but rather to help create a matrix whereby you could acquire the same accomplishments for yourself. The way to achieve appropriate goals must be unique to each of you, as individual as your separate talents, values, and desires. If you attempt to copy a path, it will be dishonest for you, and you will fail. It is in the act of searching for your path that you will grow. Please read my story just as *one example* of how goals can be achieved. More important than any financial success was my discovery that, after I had achieved every financial goal I had imagination enough to set, I found myself *miserable!* I was miserable in dentistry as well as in many other facets of my life. I had spent many years setting and achieving goals and had invested so much of who I was in their pursuit. It wasn't until I had attained so grandly that panic set in. I realized the goals I had set and had believed in all my life contained little peace or joy. Yet in this very personal misery was the seed of joy and the force that launched a deeper search for true meaning and peace in my life. While your answers and your journey will be different than mine, I hope my story may serve to guide you on your own unique path.

I sincerely desire that you understand and follow my plans for financial independence. When you achieve these goals, and during the time you are striving to reach them, I'd like your life to be joyful! Financially independent, joyful, and dentist? Which of those terms doesn't seem to fit? Let's see if we can correctly respond to that question with answer (d): they all do!

Let's begin our sojourn with a little history. For this book to be of benefit to you, you must have complete faith in my veracity. For such trust to develop you must first know who I am. For the sake of our particular mission here, we can pick up my "life story" in 1964, as I entered the University of Iowa. I was 17 years old and the oldest of five kids. Dad worked in a factory, and Mom had returned to teaching school a few years before, after a series of part-time jobs that supplemented her full-time motherhood "career." I remember filling out financial aide papers for the University of Iowa. We proudly realized that in 1963 our aggregate family income exceeded $5,000 for the first time! (That stellar financial accomplishment owed thanks to Dad having a night job at a gas station too.)

My folks loved me. They wanted very much for me to succeed. However, if I was to succeed in college, the financial obligations of that formidable task were to be entirely mine. There just didn't exist the family financial assets needed to help me through school.

Luckily, my parents had given me a gift of more value than mere money. Somehow I had always known I would go to college. I also "always" knew that getting the money was my responsibility. I doubt I was born with this awareness, but the sureness of that knowledge never left me. In the tough years that followed it was like an unfailing beacon. A vision that confirmed my true destination, that of a college graduate, no matter how dark the night.

Have you given your children this gift? Do *all* of them possess it? I put money away for my kids' education almost the moment they were born (we'll discuss the Uniform Gift to Minors Act in great detail later, and how this money has grown tax free for them). Two of my children are in college now. Both are honor students, and we anticipate years of post graduate training (not to mention expense!) in their future. But the most visible manifestation of my parents' gift occurred a short while ago, when my then–10-year-old said, "Daddy, doesn't everyone go to college?" Did this statement show arrogance on her part? Perhaps it indicates a lack of sensitivity for the "less fortunate" on her part? To me, this was a glimpse of the vision that my parents had given to me. At age 10 she possessed that same guiding beacon (in addition to money already put away to pay for her dream)! College, to her, was just a natural progressive step in her life. A task to be completed in its due time as surely as high school is.

But let's return to my story. Even at age 17, I was not without resources. I had saved money from a paper route for three years before launching a "real" career at age 13, working at a local harbor and marina. The starting pay was $0.35 per hour, but I "got" to work 70 hours a week (if you're curious how you work 70 hours, in my case it was simple: 10 hours a day seven days a week). By the time I entered the University of Iowa, I had $3,000 saved in the bank (and an as-yet-undiagnosed case of mononucleosis).

I was a pre-med major, as I'd guess were many of you. I have no idea why I chose that particular major. It did seem to help me get dates. I needed all the help I could get! I wore white socks all the time and didn't shower all that often. All the clothes I owned fit really well in my one borrowed suitcase. I remember how embarrassed I was when the maid in our dormitory told me to sleep *between* the sheets. I was used to just having one on my bed! I had graduated from high school third in my class. That would be a little more impressive if there hadn't been only 22 pupils in the class, with only four planning to go on to further formal education. Well, I think you get the picture. It's not one of sophistication, class, and confidence. When I left for the University of Iowa, I didn't know if I'd last a week.

My grades were pretty good for a working student. About a 3.3 or so. During my college years I held jobs in a power plant (assistant janitor), in a sawmill (My major efforts here revolved around trying not to be dismembered by a saw for three months. Many of the people I worked with weren't that lucky. I saw an earlobe and finger "lost" that summer.), in hay fields, as a prison guard, laboratory assistant (truth be told, I cleaned a lot of animal cages), gas jockey at a filling station, and campus policeman. All high paying and high-intellect positions, as I'm sure you can see.

By 1968 I was a university senior with no major. Service in Viet Nam was a very real and very scary possibility! As a matter of fact, as a campus policeman I got to be on the side of law and order two consecutive years, when student riots closed the entire university. I was delighted that (1) I didn't get hurt, and (2) I didn't have to take final exams when the protests were successful in closing the university both years. The main observation I was able to make at that point in my life was that it looked like a lot more fun to be on the hippie, free love, and peace side of the lines than it was where I stood, in a hot policeman's uniform.

But that's getting a little ahead of our story. In my junior year, I had abandoned pre-med to follow my true scholarly love, history. I was relatively talented in this area. Getting all A's in history was easy, especially after chemistry and physics. Then my ever-practical dad asked me a question that changed my life: what was I planning to do once I had obtained my degree in history? That shows how little some fathers understand what the college experience is all about! Of course, what really bugged me was the fact that I had no idea what I was going to do! So it's the last semester of my senior year, and I'm having an innocent soft drink at the Student Union when I run into an old dormitory buddy I haven't seen in years. He's in dental school! Weird. He says it's pretty easy, and I should give it a look. As fate (?) would have it, the dental school was right across the street from the Union. I walked over, and 15 minutes later I'm talking to a representative about the college. We have a nice visit, and he says, "While you're here, do you want to fill out an application for admission?" Why not? That was Thursday.

Two days later I received my final acceptance into dental school. It seems that doctor I talked to was the dean in charge of admissions. The final class selection took place that very evening. Our innocent visit was my interview. (Talk about low pressure. I'd have been a nervous wreck, and would probably even have showered and shaved had I known!) I took the admission test the following summer, and when they saw those results (my chalk carving wasn't too inspiring), the powers that be at the dental college may have had second thoughts. However, by then my draft board had granted my professional deferment, and I was a brand-new member of the class of 1972, University of Iowa, College of Dentistry.

The next four years masqueraded as eternity. As my chalk carving indicated, my hands weren't great. The studying wasn't too difficult, but the clinical courses were the first endeavors I had ever attempted that I couldn't perform well, no matter how hard I labored. It was during my semester of carving wax teeth that the word frustration took on a whole new meaning in my life.

I know it was different for some of you, but dental school was no fun for me. College had been a lot of work and worry, but had also been filled with the rewards of accomplishments and the support of instructors for jobs well done. Looking back to my dental school years, I'm ashamed that I allowed myself to be treated in the manner I was by a large number of the faculty. I guess I didn't fit their image of what a dental student should be. I certainly didn't know how to dress, act, or say the proper thing. I wasn't even comfortable around people who could. My work ethic and relative intelligence didn't seem to impress the dental instructors who held my fate in their hands.

I married my college sweetheart after the completion of my fifth year at the University of Iowa. I had three years of college left to finish, and Joann had one year remaining to complete her medical technology degree. Her parents offered to help us financially. I refused. I was poor, but stupid. I doubt it ever occurred to me that my wife might not like living in the dump of a Quonset hut (built during World War II to serve as temporary housing) we occupied for three years. Our humble abode did have one certain grace: the rent was $68 per month including all utilities. In the winter, it also had permanent ice *inside* the bedroom walls, where the mildew was the worst. My in-laws took one look at our truly humble abode and offered to buy us a house which they would retain as a rental property investment after we graduated. Well, I already told you I didn't know how to act around gracious people. I said no.

My junior year we were blessed with the arrival of John, Jr. We weren't blessed with medical insurance. No problem, I just worked as a campus policeman 40 hours a week, went to my 40 hours of classes, did a little studying, some eating, and very little sleeping. I doubt I was a lot of fun to be with, but the doctor got his money at the same time we got John, Jr. Could we have gotten free care as indigents? They don't get more indigent than we were! Did I even consider the option? Not really. I guess I'm just not too smart.

But I could handle 100-hour work weeks and three hours of sleep a night. I was young, and many of you probably made as great a sacrifice. What I don't understand is the abusive and negative attitude so prevalent among most of my clinical instructors. I finished dental school $4,000 in debt and exhausted. That was my choice. I also finished with a broken spirit and a deeply wounded psyche. That, to a large extent, was the faculty's choice.

How many physical and mental problems, failed marriages, and untold other pain eventually occurs as a result of emotional trauma inflicted by this group of often-unhappy individuals? (Two of our instructors attempted suicide; one succeeded. This must qualify them as unhappy. Those poor souls were two of the teachers I liked!) I've tried, in my small way, to help later dental students. I taught one semester at my alma mater and did my best to treat each student with respect and dignity. I've had five senior students grace our office for five to six weeks as preceptors before this wonderful program was abandoned by the university. In 1991 I offered to teach practice management at the dental college, *pro bono* (for free). My offer was turned down flatly and repeatedly by the Dean and a number of his factotums. Instead of accepting my services, they offered no practice management course at all! They still don't like me, I guess.

If you agree with my estimation of conditions at dental schools, what have you done to make them better? Do you understand that these current students are your brothers and sisters? Who do you think will come to their aid if we don't?

I did graduate and volunteered to enter the Army in 1972. Maybe it was a coincidence, but one month after I enlisted, American troops withdrew from Viet Nam. (It may also have been an accurate assessment by our military as to what effect my entrance into the armed service would have. They may have decided to get out while they still could.)

My two years in the service were great! I read (some of the dental texts I didn't have time to peruse as a working student), learned from some excellent and warm-hearted military dentists, and worked hard. I received *honors!* We were all dressed alike now, (in the nature of full disclosure, I must confess I look good in a drab green), and even in the military (the mother of all waste), solid effort was recognized and rewarded. (I served with a young dentist who had graduated from Ohio State a year before I left Iowa. He told me he had thrown up every morning of his last year in dental school. Doctors could find no problem. When he graduated the problem stopped. I hope and pray he's well today and not another victim of the dental school system.)

Our second child, Heather Jean, was born in Ft. Lewis, Washington, where we served our two-year military obligation. We were now rich on a salary of $16,000 a year. I had saved enough money the summer before I entered the service (by working as a dentist in the office of an established practice while the owner toured Europe) to pay off all my school debts. (I speak to young dentists today with $100,000 in student-loan debt. We'll discuss debt at length. I'm horrified at the plight of these kids. There may be a way out from under this mountain of debt for them, but the path surely isn't going to be either quick or easy. I don't want to be hard hearted, but I see this amount of school debt as an example of "buying" something that you haven't earned the right to as yet that seems so epidemic in our society.)

Now as proud and compensated members of our national defense, we bought a TV and had company visit from back home. I worked out and felt good. The positive feedback and 40-hour work weeks were my tonic. Soon we began to search for a place to establish my dental practice and build our futures.

Jo, myself, John, and baby Heather spent a total of four weeks leave time and flew back to Iowa twice in our pursuit of the perfect practice location. My mom and dad babysat our little family while we explored most of the highway in our native Iowa. Hundreds of phone calls were made. About a dozen practices were evaluated. Finally we chose a little town on the banks of the Mississippi River: Keokuk, Iowa. The dentists were relatively few, and many of them were older. All were very busy. Most were also very friendly. I liked the new YMCA; Jo, the new mall. We both liked the size of the town, about 13,000. We rented a two-bedroom upstairs apartment and located an "open office space" (so open that the floors were dirt and no inside walls had yet been built).

Our location now painstakingly selected, we began drawing office designs, calling contractors, and worrying a lot. I worked on an office practice manual for hours. In July we left the army and arrived in Keokuk. On August 18, 1974, we began seeing patients. I had hired a staff of two. (Neither had any dental experience, but they were both cute!) The first day of my private practice life we saw only people with toothaches and produced $200. Was I proud! We had begun!

Maybe this is the first critical point in our story. Those of you who wish to achieve wealth, please read what follows with care. We constructed our office for about $30,000. That total included everything from dental equipment to remodeling to paper clips. Several of the area dentists visited the office and shook their heads. They told me that I didn't need anything this nice! (Please remember, this was 1974. I spent $40,000 on an office computer system two years ago, and our last van had a $31,000 sticker on the window. Times do change!) My beloved Grandpa Kehr loaned us $10,000. We had saved about the same amount during our two years in the military. (We saved this money because we chose not to spend it. This is a pivotal concept you must comprehend. Our saving $10,000 on two-years' salary of $32,000 was a choice, not a lucky happenstance!)

For you math majors, we still had $10,000 of debt left to pay on our $30,000 investment. I had talked to the area banks before I selected Keokuk. They were very receptive and willing to helping us. I intended to approach them for a loan when all the bills had arrived and I knew the exact amount of funds we would require to complete our office. The bills trickled in, and we simply paid them with cash generated from treating patients. I worked a 6-day, 55-hour week. In March of 1975, seven months after I opened my business, Grandpa Kehr got his $10,000 back from a very proud, and not-nearly-grateful-enough, grandson. The practice was ours, free and clear.

Is this perhaps a fairy tale or an old legend from another time? Is it possible to do such a thing today? All I can testify to for sure is that I did precisely what I have just stated. Do I expect everybody to do the same? Not at all. I'm telling you this story for two reasons. Remember, as you read this book, that I want you to get to know me. To really know who I am, how I came to be, and what I believe in. Secondly, this story is an important part of my unique blueprint. You could say that the establishment of a debt-free office is the epicenter of our financial well-being blueprint.

My point is not that this is what everyone must do to be financially successful, but that this is an example of delayed gratification that may prove instructive to you. A more germane question at this juncture would be: If I desire to buy a BMW, how might my decision be affected by this story? The answer is that a choice to purchase your longed-for BMW is consistent with the philosophy of my story if you can write a check for the car (not the down payment, but for the full price of the car), if you owe no debt and have a large retirement plan funded, and also if you are certain that this or any purchase will bring you real joy. If this doesn't describe you, then I'd suggest you put off purchasing that BMW until you've actually earned it.

Please allow an example of wanting before earning from my dental experience. A staff member asked to meet with me in my private office after work. She informed me that she needed more money. She explained that some extra expenses had arisen, and she needed more income to meet these additional obligations. After patiently hearing her out, I asked her what she intended to do to make herself more valuable to the office. She seemed stunned by my question. I attempted to explain that, to me, she was asking to have before she had become. This is like the old parable about a man standing before the fireplace. His request? Give me heat, and then I will give you wood. As ridiculous as this example seems, my staff member's request was more absurd. She asked for "heat" (i.e., more money), and didn't even promise "more wood" later (i.e., greater office contributions).

I'd like to report a happy ending. Possibly an epiphany, as she discovered her request inadvertently violated her own values, which said, "Earn what you get out of life." Unfortunately this young lady had approached me with a need for more money, not more philosophy! Sadly, perhaps, she got neither.

A silly story about a young lady? But many doctors of my acquaintance have told me basically the same thing. That they need more income. That they *desire* the added revenue greatly. What they lack is any concept of a need to create more value in themselves first. It is possible to have more income without creating more value in yourself (bank robbery comes to mind), but I know of no way to accomplish this goal that is consistent with my personal values. To paraphrase a famous commercial, if you want more, obtain it the old-fashion way: *earn it!* Thus the way to have more is to become more.

I have one last parable of self-revelation to share with you here: the parable of the house. Once the office was paid for, we felt free to look for a home. (If you reasoned that four people living in a two-bedroom upstairs apartment was excellent motivation for attaining the financial ability to afford a home, I would compliment you on your perceptiveness.)

Jo and I found a new home in the country we both loved and moved in on May 30, 1975. The house cost about $42,000. We had been able to save $12,000 in the three months since Grandpa's loan was repaid. We borrowed the remaining $30,000 from my generous in-laws. Now that I knew I could repay a loan (based on nine months of steadily rising income), I was able to accept their help. We paid this loan back fully within three years. At this point, with an office, car, and home owned free and clear (I love that phrase) at the age of 31, it was time to begin saving in earnest! But much more on that later.

One last legacy learned in my childhood: It's fine to go without. It is not fine to have what you don't deserve. If you don't have the money to purchase something, then you don't deserve to possess it. If you must go into debt, at least know that in doing so you now possess something that you as yet haven't earned the right to. Make every effort to become worthy as rapidly as possible. My education, office, and home were the only three investments for which I ever borrowed money. There will be no fourth one.

Today we have savings of over $1,400,000, all in cash, bonds, and quality stocks. (This doesn't include the value of my home, office, etc, which you know I own debt free.) We owe no one. Am I proud and bragging? You bet! But I hope you see the real issue. Nobody started much lower than I, yet, by the time I had achieved age 40 (born December 14, 1946), I had $1,000,000 in savings. Dentistry in Keokuk, Iowa (well-known hotbed of dental excellence), did this for me. I have never had another source of income.

For the past four years I have worked eight days a month, or 100 days a year. My earned income before taxes is about $200,000 annually. I make almost $100,000 a year more from investment returns. I didn't make fabulous investments with huge rates of return. All my investments are safe, conservative, and thus lower in rate of return. I sure as hell didn't inherit anything. *The path that got me here is open to each and every one of you,* even if you aren't fortunate enough to practice in that dental Mecca of Keokuk, Iowa. Few of you will have trouble matching my skills as a clinician (a larger number would laugh at them). I promise you that as vital as clinical excellence is to dental success, the least skilled of us, with hard work and dedication, can achieve a level of technical expertise that will allow all our dreams to be fulfilled.

Before this book is finished, I will have shared with you a lot of "tricks" that we have implemented to help us arrive where we are today, both in my dental practice and the financial world. But the biggest "trick" is in your personal mindset. I live a life of leisure with many choices. (The true use of money is to purchase freedom and choices, as well as a few toys along the path.) I still see patients, but only because I choose to. I have worked very hard, but I have been rewarded. This is the gift I wish to give to you: that you can see the possible in the world, and find your path to it. Also, that the path be filled with joy and meaning along the way. Often mine wasn't. But then, I didn't have this book to help guide me on my way.

CHAPTER 2

---◆---

THE KEY IS
PHILOSOPHY

This chapter is absolutely central to the message this book is attempting to convey. *Please pay your closest attention to what follows.* Sadly, I believe many in our profession feel that philosophy and psychology have no practical impact on the successful practice of dentistry. My guess would be that people who give credence to such a statement are not prospering in their dental careers and are possibly unhappy in their personal lives. Yes, a request for a serious examination of personal and professional philosophy will be met by resistance from some. Perhaps they regard the subject as of no significance to "real" dentistry. Maybe it is perceived as just plain scary. The more your tendency is to resist, the more you are in need of this message. Some will enthusiastically welcome such information. For those more-aware individuals, I hope to add a little additional insight to a subject on which they are already well informed.

Those of you who find the topic of philosophy foreign and disturbing may wish to hurry on to the how-to-make-money part, which seems grounded more comfortably in what is perceived to be reality.

Please don't leave us now. The "hard facts" contained in other sections of this book *may* show you how to create more wealth, but the fragmented tips you pick up from such a cursory review of this book won't show you how to attain joy. And make no mistake, joy is the goal. Money is merely a byproduct, created in the process of attaining your bliss. A congruent personal philosophy is the matrix that holds all these threads of information together as one solid fabric. Using the facts in this book without such a matrix would be like trying to clothe yourself with threads. While not impossible, it would certainly be an impractical way to fashion daily attire.

The simple truth: We don't really have a choice of being or not being a psychologist or philosopher. We do have a choice of being consciously aware of our philosophy of life and attempting to maximize the benefits a congruent, well-thought-out philosophy can achieve for us or to ignore the task of clearly defining our own philosophy and suffer the consequences of letting critical decisions in our lives be decided on whim and whimsy. Thus our choice is between intelligently using philosophy to improve our lives and careers or ignoring the subject at our peril.

I believe part of our reluctance to deal with these critical subjects that offer such tremendous opportunities to enrich our lives is a combination of genetic selection and training. We in dentistry are people of science. If we weren't, we wouldn't have been accepted into dental school, much less have been able to successfully complete that rigorous course of training. This means that due to our inherent nature, our training, or both, we have a predilection for "hard facts." You may wish to debate whether people of science are born or created. Whatever your decision, I believe you'll agree that the great majority of us involved in the practice of dentistry are scientists.

Such a strong bias toward the scientific would be more efficacious if we lived in a world where every question had a clear and factual answer. I guess such a place would be a world with no people, possibly containing only computers. Our world teems with such messy subjects as people, their feelings, and judgments, where often no absolute "right answer" exists. In such a world we are forced, no matter our level of comfort, to deal with such inexact subjects as emotion and philosophy.

The literature on right- and left-brain function is extensive. If you aren't well informed on this subject, you have some badly needed remedial work to accomplish. Understanding this concept is essential to function maximally in the world we inhabit. For our discussion's sake, let's simply say that the left hemisphere of the brain controls our rational and verbal functions. The right hemisphere is the nonverbal feeling part of the brain. We receive communication from this hemisphere in pictures, dreams, or visions. All of us have and use both cerebral sections, but some of us function with much greater comfort in one hemisphere than in the other. We have a strong tendency to function in the hemisphere where we are most comfortable and to view people who tend to function with a different hemispheric orientation than our own with suspicion and distrust.

Mr. Spock, of *Star Trek* fame, is the quintessential representation of a fully left-brain person. No emotion is possible for him, only logic. Most of the old TV series showed how Captain Kirk constantly solved problems his brilliant friend Spock couldn't solve or comprehend. Captain Kirk's secret weapon was to draw on the seeming weakness of human emotions to overcome his interplanetary difficulties. (I hope all "trekkers" will allow this gross oversimplification in order to establish a point.)

In literature at least, the dominant right-brain characters tend to be female. Scarlet O'Hara, of *Gone With the Wind* fame, simply dismissed painful reality by stating that she would think about it tomorrow. Her solution to the problems of life was to ignore situations that were unpleasant for her. She simply dismissed from her awareness realities that she disliked and chose to live in a world consistent with her concept of what reality should be. Such unpleasantness as the Civil War and the loss of the person she loved most were put aside until tomorrow.

I guess most of us, from time to time, copy Scarlet's philosophy of ignoring unpleasant reality in the hopes it will go away. An example of such behavior from my life would be not dismissing an employee badly in need of an "expansion of employment opportunity," with the hope that his/her behavior would somehow magically improve. While not as extreme as ignoring a war swirling all about me, this is still an example from the head-in-the-sand school of dental practice management. How nice life would be, if by simply waiting, all of our problems would solve themselves. Having personal extensive experience with this approach, I hope you will trust me when I tell you: It didn't work for Scarlet, it hasn't worked for me, and worst of all, it isn't going to work for you.

If Mr. Spock were a practicing dentist, he would deal with "just the facts." He would be uncomfortable and confused by people around him that suffered from such strange afflictions as anxiety (never say fear to a dentist), sadness, or anger. I'm sure Dr. Spock would be excellent at diagnosis, but I don't think he'd be a lot of fun to work for, and I doubt you'd have to wait too long for an appointment to be seen in his office. We humans all have feelings and are more comfortable around other people (even dentists) who are aware and comfortable with their own emotional states.

These are two fictitious examples of extreme hemisphere imbalance. Both Scarlet and Mr. Spock are characterizations of people functioning almost totally in one mode, either logic or emotion, to the point of denying reality. No such total separation is possible in real life, only a tendency to one extreme or the other. My concern is that in dentistry I see many practitioners who are very uncomfortable with their emotions.

Are you uncomfortable making decisions you can't prove to be right? Maybe you sometimes avoid making any commitment, so you can escape all possibilities of being wrong. It's safer for you to let someone else make key management decisions, from collection policies to the way you dress for work.

Does it bother you if someone else cries? Do you feel it is wrong to be sad, angry, or otherwise experience feelings? These are signs of discomfort with right hemisphere function. Said another way, such behaviors indicate an attempt by individuals to *deny the functioning of their own brains*, as these particular activities don't coincide with what they perceive their own self-image "should" be.

The descriptions of possible emotion-producing situations are endless (especially in my office), but the point is, are you comfortable with *feelings?* Everyone (even dentists) has them. You can deny your feelings, which is dishonest, but you can't not have them. While we are unable to avoid having emotions, we do have choices as to how to deal with them. We can choose to be aware of the feelings and use them to understand and grow, both in our business and life. Or we can choose to deny and bottle up emotion, thus failing to use them as tools to help us learn and understand.

Whatever our choice, these denied emotions still exist. Feelings can be disguised, but even if thus rendered invisible, they continue to affect our lives on both a physical and emotional level. These repressed feelings can show up at 4 A.M., ending a needed night's rest. They may appear when you blow up for no apparent reason (possibly at some innocent victim, often a loved one). Maybe they'll show up as an ulcer, hypertension, colitis, or cancer. Whatever form emotions eventually take, denying that your feelings exist makes as much sense as walking in the rain, but assuring everyone that you're not really getting wet.

The keys to *self-understanding*, as well as personal and professional *growth*, lie within these scary feelings. We are going to discuss how to clarify values at length in the following chapter. We will demonstrate how to use the values you identify to create a consistent philosophy in your personal and professional life. This clarified philosophy provides you with all the answers for *all* the questions. Once you have precisely defined that which you deeply believe in and further clarified these beliefs by codifying them in written form, every question asked of you can be answered by referring back to this statement in your beliefs.

In our office, this statement of collective values is called *Our Purpose*. It hangs on the wall in every room of our office. We read it aloud before every staff meeting begins. Often we discuss new ideas or examine our behavior from the context of "Are our actions consistent with our purpose?" Every predicament, when examined from this perspective, has a clear and evident solution. We'll discuss the birth and continuing life of this collective office purpose shortly.

Without such a clear statement of our collective beliefs, many decisions would be made on the basis of the feelings of the moment. Often this mood is the result of an accidental juxtaposition of several random events, such as too many grumpy people encountered in a row. A critical decision may be made based on the level of our blood sugar or adrenaline at that particular moment. Maybe, while in a "good mood," we make a commitment that will prove difficult to keep over the long haul. Perhaps, while in a "bad mood," we pass up what could have proven to be a golden opportunity.

Such a random decision-making technique (or lack of same) is akin to everyone on board a cruise ship taking turns steering at random intervals. Our purpose acts as our map and compass, first to chart a path to our desired destination and then to be referred to constantly, to assure us that we are indeed still on our chosen course.

Emotions are the keys that guide us to discover our true identities. The feelings that you possess must be identified, examined, and understood. Only then can they become our allies in a quest for a more complete and happier existence. We often become so adept at covering up our feelings that it is hard even for us to accurately identify them. In some ways this covering of feelings may be helpful. An example could be when you have just finished a difficult procedure with a result that's not all you'd hoped for. You are less than completely collected, yet you must go on to care for another patient. To display your emotion to that patient wouldn't be fair to him or her or very professional of you. But we must remember that the feelings remaining from the upsetting incident still exist, even if we have chosen to ignore them for the moment. The danger inherent in this situation is that we grow so out of touch with our own feelings as to believe the emotions no longer exist. By choosing to block our own perception of our emotional states, we risk losing the ability to accurately identify your emotions when it is appropriate and useful to do so.

Allow me to illustrate this point by using a painful example from my own life. In this incident my tendency to bury my feelings and the level of skill I had achieved at denying my feelings existed were revealed to me in a stunning and graphic manner.

When my daughter Megan was five, she suffered a skull fracture that resulted in a bruising of the brain. She was unconscious for several days. During these nightmarish days and nights while Megan remained comatose, a wise friend asked me how I felt. I described Megan's injury. She replied, "I asked you how *you felt*." I then described my actions of the last few days. She wouldn't quit. She said, "You're not hearing my question. Pretend that Megan is right here with us now, lying on the floor in front of you. What would you like to tell her?" It wasn't until I visualized Megan lying there with us, that I realized how terrified I was.

After I identified my true feelings, things got easier. I no longer had to pretend. There is great freedom in honesty, while pain and loss of energy result from attempted self-deceit. Megan woke up after three days, and fully recovered. In some ways, I never did, because little about me remained unchanged from that experience, now some six years in the past. Somewhere during that period of time, perhaps as I sat up all night to be certain Megan wouldn't aspirate the clear fluid she vomited, I lost my ability to pretend that my feelings didn't exist.

I had been forced to look at the reality of my own emotions, a thing I had avoided at all costs for quite a while. In my drive for what I perceived to be success, I had no time for puny emotions. I simply froze them and moved on. I was an irresistible force, brooking no impedance on my path to "success."

All the things that a moment prior to Megan's injury had seemed so critically important to me were almost instantly reevaluated. In some areas of my life I now felt as exposed as a newborn chick, fresh from my protective shell of closed-off emotions. This seeming protection from the pain of life is the payoff we believe we receive when our emotions are denied. In exchange for this numbness we give up our chance for growth and true happiness.

To summarize to this point: Our only choices in the matter of philosophy are to be aware of the crucial importance it plays in our lives and to choose to use philosophy constructively to bring us wisdom, success, and joy or to ignore its place as a central factor in our existence and suffer the painful consequences that a random pattern of decision-making in our life will create. Those without a clearly defined philosophy are the dentists I speak to that wish to attain great wealth one day, to be a charity worker on another, to give up the profession and to live in the mountains on the third, and to take all the Pankey courses at once on the next. They are probably still considering careers as cowboys or lawyers in their leisure moments. (Personally, I have trouble separating the two last-stated professions myself, so perhaps they can be forgiven here.) They are drifting through life much as a rudderless ship. Their chances of ending up at their hoped for destination in life are about as probable as that of the unguided ship sailing into its desired port.

A key to uncovering our own personal philosophy lies in the messy, inexact realm of emotions. We must learn to identify our feelings, and grow to see *all emotions* as our friends and guides (not just the feelings we have chosen to define as pleasant). Using our awareness of these feelings, we can proceed to clarify our own values, and thus develop an accurate personal philosophy that will allow us to divine answers to some of life's questions.

We must learn to integrate both our left (logic) and right (emotion) brain functions to allow whole brain thinking. Dentistry is too tough to go through with half your brain tied behind your back (although you can make a fortune that way as a TV or radio host/author, I've been told).

I have placed my emphasis on those among us who have repressed or undeveloped right-brain function, because in our profession I believe the dental-school selection process and the curriculum of the dental college itself have done a wonderful job of eliminating people lacking in left brain ability. This system has created a "survival of the fittest" scenario that eliminates right brainers in a manner that even Darwin never envisioned.

For those of you so inclined, the process of developing whole-brain integrated function is the Hero's quest. A clear philosophy—and its use in our lives—is the Holy Grail we seek. Armed with this prize, we can better serve our own needs, and those of our fellow men. This is the universal story in most of the great myths of mankind. In a myth, a clarified personal philosophy may be symbolized as a golden fleece, the discovery of fire, or a pot of gold. Don't be mislead by these disguises: a philosophy of life that benefits us and our fellow men is always the true prize sought. As with most deep truths, the process is fairly simple to comprehend. It is not, however, easy to accomplish!

Ask yourself, What is your Holy Grail? What do you want most from the abundance this world offers? Is it riches, joy, peer approval, or love? Whatever your choice, you can attain it. The methods by which you may obtain your desires will be explained in this very book. You need only read it with discernment. By becoming comfortable with your emotions and using them to identify your true values, when you do achieve your goals, they will be truly yours and will contain joy.

A wise man once advised to be careful of what you set your heart to, for surely you shall get it. Please take this stark warning seriously. Little in this world impacts as sharply as achievement of a long-held dream, only to find it contains no real happiness or meaning for you.

CHAPTER 3

VALUE
CLARIFICATION

Value clarification is simply the task of identifying what we truly believe in. Be warned: It is not the task of identifying what we have been told we should believe in or identifying what we wished we believed in. Assuredly, the process is difficult and never-ending, yet I know of no exercise which returns as large a dividend in terms of added joy and success in your life for your efforts. The method I use to clarify my own values is threefold:

STEP 1. Spend a lot of time thinking. It seems in our culture today that quiet thought is a dreaded thing, to be avoided at all cost by many. Do you tend to have the TV or radio on when you're alone? What is it you wish to avoid in your own thoughts? Do you like to be around people or to be busy all the time? From what force do you seek to flee? Peace and solitude in a location that is your quiet place are what's needed to achieve a better understanding of yourself, to find authentic solutions to life's troubles and mysteries. This quiet place can be the library, your own office when no one else is around, or a room at home where you will seldom be disturbed. I have a basement study that is my quiet place of sanctuary.

Obtain such a place for yourself, whatever the cost. The only other requirements needed for this exercise are a pen and paper to record your thoughts and, if you like, a hot cup of coffee. Think deeply and often about who you are and what you believe. Set aside a regular time, at least 30 minutes for this task only, at least once a week. *Do nothing else* during this special time! Your mind will wander; such is the nature of minds. It's very tempting to reflect on topics more interesting and safer than self-discovery. My favorite alternative topic is how messed up *other* people are. This is indeed much more entertaining, but unfortunately will not help you grow as a person or prove helpful to those you are reflecting upon. (At least the people with whom I've been compassionate enough to share my perceptions of the problems that exist in their lives have never returned to thank me for my thoughtful assistance. Now that I think about it, they often don't even return.)

With persistence, this task of quiet reflection will become easier. Just continue to redirect your mind to concerns that deal with you alone. The daydreaming and loss of focus on the desired topic will lessen as fear of examining your feelings and beliefs decreases. Productive ideas will soon fill your note pad, each thought a potential gem in value. Is it time to add an associate, chairside, or hygienist? How can you best deal with your son's earring or daughter's purple hair? The one difficulty I have *never* had to confront is having no problems in my life to deal with.

STEP 2. Observe your own behavior. As the day goes by, and most especially at the end of the day as you drift off to sleep, review your behavior and your emotions from the day. Bravely identify both those events which caused you pain, as well as those that brought you joy. The secret to happiness is to do a lot of the activities that bring joy and to avoid those which cause pain and don't help you to grow. Simple, but not easy.

If you fail to notice and identify the joy and pain, it's impossible to systematically increase the joyful, while decreasing the painful. *Awareness* is the vital first step to meaningful change. Don't fall into the traps of false joy, taking drugs, overeating, cheating on your spouse: In time these transient pleasures will result in long-term pain. Concentrate on true happiness. You may find real joy in such mundane things as patience shown or a kind word given or received. You must develop the ability to see through the short term and observe that which creates true, long-term pleasure.

For instance, do you hate every day when you are scheduled to remove a tooth? I do. I spent a lot of years removing a lot of teeth. I took courses and studied exodontia, thinking that as my skills improved, so would my enjoyment, or at least comfort, with the procedures. Despite my honest efforts, my feelings toward tooth removals stayed negative. I no longer remove teeth. Instead I concentrate on preforming the procedures I enjoy. Maybe unpleasantness for you involves certain types of patients: perhaps the very old or very young. Perhaps it's molar endodontics that makes you cringe to see on the day's schedule. Maybe it's a member of your own staff that day after day diminishes your joy. Identify the pain and move from it. Find a way to create joy in the situation. (Maybe you can discuss your concerns with your staff member. Perhaps taking a course on endodontics could help.) If you can't find a way for this painful situation to bring you joy, my advice is concise: Remove the offending situation from your life. A bumper sticker I saw in Colorado sums this philosophy up nicely: "Life is too short to dance with ugly people."

Would you live with a cancer because it paid you rent? Will you continue *choosing* to suffer pain to obtain money? Or is the cause of your suffering your own fear of change? Clarifying your values will help here. I doubt life without pain is a possibility (at least not until we shuffle off this mortal coil). What I believe to be possible is to minimize pain and also to deliberately decide when you will choose to accept unpleasantness, because the painful episode is part of a process that will, once endured, lead you to personal growth. If you want joy, move from pain. Do you wish financial independence? Does debt or a lack of money cause you concern? Identify that which brings you wealth, and do more of it. Identify that which reduces wealth, and do less of that. When you choose to spend, be certain that the purchase is consistent with your values and not just the result of some transitory emotion. If you won't do these things, then your choice is clear: learn to find joy in poverty. At least accept the fact that poverty is your choice, a product of your collective decision-making in this area of your life and not something forced on you by sinister outside powers.

STEP 3. Observe and modify your values by awareness of your feelings. The behaviors of others that make you feel uncomfortable contain the seeds of great knowledge. Their actions which leave you upset, illustrate the parts of yourself with which you are not yet at peace. Let's take one hypothetical example of behavior in others you dislike and see how you can grow from observing it.

Do you hate cheap behavior in others? Then come to grips with the frugal part of yourself, and try to understand why it distresses you. Has someone told you that to be cheap is bad? Has the image of yourself as a free spender conflicted with a dislike of waste? It's not good or bad to spend money. This action is simply a choice you make. *Our feelings tell us how close our choice of behavior is to what our true values really are.* It is painful to have no clear guidelines as to our personal philosophy concerning the use of money. One day you are a consumer, the next a saver. Each action frustrating the other. As is always the case, *unclear values cause confusion and pain.*

Allow me another illustration. Are you uncomfortable with displays of anger by others? Then you're uncomfortable with your own feelings of anger. No amount of self-control can eliminate your anger, only disguise it. Emotions are not bad or good, they simply are. Use these emotional windows of insight to study your own makeup. The things you hate are parts of yourself that you have yet to accept. You have condemned them as evil, based on what is undoubtably incomplete knowledge internalized at an early age. Take these uncomfortable feelings out of the prison of unacceptable behavior you have consigned them to and restore them once again as an acceptable segment of who you are, a part whose purpose and duty you understand and respect, even if you don't admire it greatly. Without the use of these parts of your personality, *you are incomplete as a person.* Another way to employ feelings to help us mature is to observe our own behavior more perceptively. What are the true feelings, both positive and negative, that certain situations create in you? Examine and identify your emotions carefully, because these feelings can guide you in the choice of behaviors that will be most efficacious for you to select in the future.

Are the feelings you have appropriate for the situation, or do they reflect childhood memories that aren't an accurate representation of existing reality? Feelings that may have been helpful, even important at age four, may no longer be helpful to us today. Only by carefully examining our behavioral choices and our emotions can decisions concerning the helpfulness and correctness of our current emotional states be reached.

I have always been uncomfortable with conflict. My tendency is to simply avoid it. I now realize that often conflict can be helpful in the growth process. As you'll see later, in our staff meetings we use communication exercises that deliberately draw out conflicting feelings. I still don't like conflict, but I am comfortable enough with it to no longer feel a need to avoid it, and thus can choose to use conflict constructively for my personal growth.

Maybe as a child, anger was an effective behavioral choice for you to employ in dealing with your parents, friends, or siblings. Perhaps it gave you control and thus comfort in difficult situations. Is it helpful for you today if you blow up at work? Does frequent staff turnover or loss of patients from your tantrums indicate that you now need to examine this behavior to see if it is still appropriate? There may be times, such as in a racquetball game, where anger can be productive and create needed energy that can be constructively channelled. In the afore-mentioned office situations, it may be inappropriate and counterproductive. You have the power to observe your behavior, to review the results, and to plan whatever changes you feel are indicated to achieve the outcomes you desire. Such behavioral awareness is called mastery.

It is not appropriate to feel shame or guilt as a failure in life because you were less than perfect at any given moment. Shame is a feeling we experience when we perceive ourselves not as people who acted badly, but as *bad people*. It is a feeling of utter devastation and helplessness. I suspect such an emotion often precedes suicide. Such feelings cause pain without allowing us an opportunity for growth. If you suffer from similar feelings, they are probably reactions from very early in your life. Freeing yourself from these destructive, but traditional emotional reactions will be very difficult, but it must be done if you wish to have joy and peace in your life. It can be helpful to feel badly about your behavior. Therein lie the seeds of positive change. It is not helpful nor accurate to feel you are a bad person with no hope of change. A condition of hopeless shame never truly exists, but is simply an error in our perception.

The first necessary step which will allow us to grow by using the information available from our own feelings is to identify exactly what emotion you are feeling. It takes both time and real effort for most of us to clearly label fear, tension, or slight apprehension. With attention and practice you will soon be able to quickly identify what physical sensations in your body are related to which emotion. How does fear feel in your stomach? In your muscles? Imagine or remember a fearful situation. Try to identify the physical manifestations of that state you were in at a later time. Repeat the exercise with anger, frustration, and any other emotional responses of which you are aware.

Next, examine the appropriateness of your feelings. Some unpleasant emotions are earned by behavior on your part that doesn't coincide with your values. The discomfort caused by acting in a way inconsistent with values we hold deeply can guide us to more appropriate behavior in the future and thus make our life more productive and happy. Said another way, when we behave badly, we need to feel badly. This discomfort, if we don't ignore it, is our guide and mentor that pushes us to reexamine the behavior that caused this pain and leads us to create a better plan of action for the next similar situation.

I have days when I seemed dogged by a feeling of uneasiness. Usually this unpleasantness is accompanied by fatigue. It's only with great effort that I can continue through the day. If I take a moment, I can identify a particular event that initiated the feelings. Maybe I didn't take the time to really do my best. Perhaps I spoke sharply to a patient or staff member, and now I'm subconsciously aware of my remorse. The error may be correctable. Simply saying "I'm sorry" can make several people feel instantly better. It may be a situation I can learn from. Perhaps I should have rescheduled to finish the endo, or even referred that particular patient. Sometimes I find that I did all that I could, and my negative feelings are unfair to me and after careful consideration, should be dismissed.

Whatever the result, the time involved is a few minutes at most. The result a much more pleasant day for myself and for all those around me. If I choose not to reflect, I get to carry these feelings like a bag full of snakes throughout the day and into the night. Which choice seems best to you? A few moments of quiet reflection to consider your past behavior and to grow, or taking the snakes home with you?

We can also mature by identifying emotions, such as shame and guilt, that cause pain but do not promote personal growth. Look back on your life and attempt to understand the origins of such feelings. Decide if these feelings can be of use in making your behavior more consistent with your values, or would best be eliminated by a better understanding of their origins and a conscious effort to be aware of why these feelings exist, and how destructive they are. As we've said, if painful feelings don't lead us to grow, we need to eliminate them. Usually this requires understanding why these feelings exist (there is always a reason), and also the awareness that the reasoning that created these painful feelings was flawed or is no longer valid. Freedom from shame and guilt releases tremendous energy that can now be used toward positive ends.

Anxiety, insomnia, headaches, and many similar disorders can be eliminated when the cause of the problem is identified and understood. Sadly, our culture has a bias to the "easy answers" and tends to prefer alcohol, sleeping pills, or destructive behavior to honest understanding and growth. Ask yourself where you tend to be in this choice of behavioral approaches. Do you tend to courageously face painful situations and acknowledge them as potential areas of personal growth, or do you hide in the world of drugs, avoidance, or the blaming of others? I like to say the choices are like taking a shower (understanding and growth) or spraying perfume over the stink (techniques that attempt to cover, but not help the problem).

SNAKES IN THE BAG

There is an Indian legend whose wisdom I often reflect on. A young brave went to the desert to seek his vision. He fasted for three days, but no vision came. On the fourth day, as he meditated, his gaze lingered on the crest of a distant snow-capped mountain. Instantly he thought, "On the top of that mountain a vision will be mine." He set out on his climb, and after a great struggle, he reached the peak. The view was inspiring! He stood in the snow and gazed in awe at the spectacle of his world revealed to him from this great height.

Suddenly, he noticed movement by his feet. It was a rattlesnake, so cold and hungry it could barely move. The snake pleaded with the boy to take him down to the desert. He knew well the danger of the snake. But at last the snake convinced him that it surely wouldn't hurt the one who saved its life.

The young brave gently picked the snake up and placed it in his bag. He set off down the mountain. When he reached the desert floor, the boy lifted the snake out and set him carefully on the warm sands. The snake coiled and struck the boy.

"How could you do this to one who has done you such a great service?" said the stunned boy.

"You knew what I was when you picked me up," replied the snake.

You got any snakes in your bag? You do if you drink to excess, use drugs, smoke, have sexual relations outside a monogamous relationship, and on and on. As I said, this story comes to mind often: when I meet a young, single girl who is pregnant or hear of a car wreck caused by speeding, or carelessness which takes the life of the driver (who wasn't wearing a seat belt). None of us, when we begin to use alcohol, smoke, use recreational drugs, or _____ (fill in the destructive behavior of your choice), is unaware of the danger. Somehow, our particular snake convinced us that *we* would be safe. In Hindu legend, one of the greatest wonders of life is that as men are dying all around, each man believes himself to be safe. Examine your life in the light of this ancient story. How does it pertain directly to you?

CLEAR VALUES

This is a dental book, but I know that you can't be a happy dentist and a miserable person. Unclear values doom you to both a personal and professional life of frustration, fear, and uncertainty. Personal value clarification must come before, or at least along with, your office value clarification. That said, let me give you an example of how value clarification changed the life of my office, myself, and my staff. Please remember that personal clarification is much more essential to your success and happiness, even if office clarification may appear less threatening.

> **Our Purpose:** Our office exists to serve the people we have dedicated ourselves to—our patients. We will create an environment of honesty and professionalism where the patient will feel comfortable, cared for, and welcome. All patients will be aware of the quality of care they receive and the sincere care of the staff for them.

We pledge to be positive, supportive team members and to create a place where we are able to have fun while encouraging and supporting personal and professional growth.

This statement of our collective values is framed and hangs in every room of our office. It took our staff a year to create this document. The reason its value is so great to us lies not in the statement itself, but in the *process that created it.* I have had visitors ask if they can copy our purpose and use it themselves. Certainly they may, but they have missed the entire point. It is the *process* of creation, not the product, that is imperative.

We began the creation of this statement with each staff member individually listing what they believed to be the central beliefs that made our office what it was. We also asked them to list what office and personal values they could identify and what behaviors we could eliminate to move us closer to what we wished our office to be. All of these ideas were committed to writing and then reviewed by one individual to eliminate duplication.

With this list in hand, we met several times as a group and discussed each point separately. Many suggested ideas were abandoned as not authentic, at least to the majority. New points were identified in these group discussions and required further exploration. In the course of this review, many office policies were immediately changed when we realized they weren't consistent with the office value core we were identifying.

At last we attempted to create one document. Each staff member wrote out their personal version of our office beliefs. All of these documents were considered and discussed. Finally, a version that we could all commit to was drafted as it appears.

None of the steps we took were critical. The discussion and not the document is the point. Each of us was helped by the candid discussions with our teammates to more clearly identify what we felt our office stood for. Each of us grew in understanding of our jobs, our fellow workers, and ourselves during the process. The value of the team grew exponentially as we identified common values and thus created a common purpose to which all were committed.

Did we make more money as a result of creating this purpose

together? Though this event took place many years ago, I'm sure we did. The truth is that positive change in our office is almost always rewarded by increased financial gain. Did we grow closer as a group? Did we grow in friendship and understanding of each other? Did we share joy in the process as well as some pain? What do you believe?

Some chose to leave our staff during this growth process. The process didn't drive them away, it just identified clearly to them that they were in the wrong place. They didn't leave in anger. They left to go to a place where the group values were closer to what they perceived their own values to be. Their leaving removed a great deal of frustration and turmoil, both in the lives of the team members who left and in those of us who remained. Once our values had been so clearly identified, the hiring of new people with similar values and beliefs was much easier.

The staff that chose to leave are still our friends. Two people can hold very different values and still like and respect each other. We wrote excellent letters of recommendation for the departing staff members, commensurate with the benefit they had given us as employees. We kept them employed until they found other work. These were good people, and it didn't take them long to find other employment, especially with our staff's assistance and support.

Over the passing years, two of the staff members who chose to leave have returned to our office family as employees. They seem to have missed the very thing that had bothered them in our office previously: the openness, honesty, and deep sense of a team mission. When they returned, their values had become very close to our own stated beliefs. I would like to think that they grew and returned as closer friends than they had been when they left.

I believe the development of an office purpose to be absolutely essential if you desire an office that produces a lot of excellent dentistry, rewards each team member financially, and creates an environment of common purpose and mutual growth. Without a clear purpose you can have some of the previously listed achievements, but you can't attain them all. Development of such a purpose requires a group of people that will commit to a difficult, at times frightening, and time-consuming process. It can not occur without a leader (that's *you*, doctor) who not only has a deep commitment to clarifying the office values, but has worked through the clarification process personally.

Let me give you the sad news straight: You can't be a wannabe and achieve this goal of value clarification in your office. This is not a task you can delegate to your faithful receptionist and expect it to be done in two weeks. The difficult task of value clarification must be under way in your life before attempting such a thing in your office, or your staff will quickly see you as a manipulative phony, trying to achieve that which hasn't been earned. Hard words, but true. To have, *you* must become. A central message of this whole book is that you can achieve whatever in life you desire, but only by personally earning it. You must first become worthy of success and then attain it.

Such a philosophy takes all the fun out of blaming others for our shortcomings. "My staff would never want to undertake a task like this; they don't have the commitment and the understanding!" Maybe you're beginning to see what they truly lack: *leadership*.

The road I'm describing is messy, inexact, and difficult. It has no end in this lifetime. The reason to embark on it is to attain joy. Is your life full of joy now? Do you share common values with your spouse? With your children? If you do, then your staff can work to create this self understanding and growth. Don't you believe such an accomplishment to be possible with all the people in your life you care enough about to make the effort for?

A world where you know exactly what you desire out of every situation. A world where you are surrounded at every turn by people who know what you believe in and share many of the same values. Think of the joy! Conflict over values (such as, Do we stay late to see emergency patients and do it cheerfully? or Do we all arrive on time for work in a proper physical and mental condition each and every day?) has been eliminated by understanding. The energy tied up in these conflicts is now ours to spend on pleasure and growth.

Put away your tendency to argue, defend yourself, and win. These needs come from your fear. Instead, confront your fear and use it to grow. Look deeply into your life and clearly see what has meaning to you. Help those dear to you to do the same, in love and not judgment. "Do the thing and have the power." Dare to create a world as you truly wish it to be.

CHAPTER 4

SELF-IMAGE

I've suffered from a low self-image, or low self-esteem, all my life. I say suffered because people who deep down don't feel good about themselves do suffer. They spend a lot of their time and energy trying to prove to others that they really are good people, worthy of respect, while never for a minute believing it themselves. They try endlessly to be "the best" (whatever that means) in an effort to get some relief from the nagging dread that at any minute everyone will find out what they're *really* like and then will avoid or laugh at them.

I first realized that self-image was a big problem in my life when I was in college. I remember the moment of epiphany when I grasped it all. I had a real sense of euphoria. Now I understood what was causing so many of my personal problems. In this flash of insight, I could clearly see what internal forces had directed most of my behavior that had caused me pain. It seemed that with this insight I had found the key to changes in my life that would result in happiness and peace. It may be so, but 20-plus years later, I'm still struggling. Understanding the dynamics of low self-esteem is a critical first step, but still only one tentative first step toward a more joyful life.

Do you have a problem with your self-image? I would guess all of us do to some extent and in some circumstances. The key to answering this question for yourself lies in an examination of your feelings. Do you often feel frightened or apprehensive for no apparent reason? One example of this type of anxiety in my life was a vague but definite uneasiness on Sundays, which got worse as the day proceeded. The feeling was not related to any behavior or circumstance, it was just there. If you step out of a cabin door and come face to face with a bear, apprehension is a reasonable and even helpful emotion. To be nervous because it's Sunday is neither reasonable, nor most likely helpful.

Do you tend to avoid new activities for fear of failing or looking foolish? Do you need to *win* at almost anything (in an effort to prove you're OK)? If you beat your kids in games or have to try hard not to, that behavior could be an insight. A vague, frequent feeling of apprehension for no clear reason, a burning need to win, and a fear of new things and situations are some of the clearest manifestations of low self-esteem in my life.

I think most of us feel insecure in some situations. It may be public speaking that tests your deodorant. Maybe it's a certain type of patient distinguished by age, behavior, or gender (i.e., perhaps you're uncomfortable with women your mom's age). It might be specific personality types that affect you. I'm very uncomfortable around a very outspoken, bossy-type person.

For each of us there are also areas of relative security where we feel in charge and comfortable. For you it may be on the golf course, at your home or office, or in any activity or place where you feel in control. My point is that our image of ourselves varies, day to day, situation to situation. How much sleep we've had, if we've been eating right, and the last encounter we experienced, pleasant or unpleasant: all can exert an effect on our self-image. Our current task is to attempt to understand where this image comes from and to create a method whereby the image of ourselves becomes as positive and productive for us in our lives as possible.

I have a theory about poor self-esteem. I think it is taught or learned at a very early age. I remember studying the concept of unconditional love in a college psychology class. I thought it was some kind of fairy tale. The idea that someone loves you no matter what your behavior was beyond my ability to grasp. I've always felt I was as good as my achievements. I guess I've always been a member of the what-have-you-done-for-me-lately? school of self-esteem. I still am reluctant to try new things because I fear "not looking good" and reinforcing my perception that I'm inadequate.

I believe today that my parents do and did have this unconditional love for me. The problem developed because what was expressed (or at least what I heard) was not "We love you, no matter what you do," but rather "You are only as good as your most recent behavior." I suppose this starts around potty training time. You are a "good boy" if you control your bodily functions. If you don't or can't, you're bad. Whatever the origins of low self-esteem, it centers around linking a person's value to their behavior. I'm sure lots of you dentists reading this right now are puzzled. "What other way is there to evaluate a person's worth than by his actions?" you may be wondering.

An infant doesn't hear "I love you as a person. You have great value to me simply by the fact that you exist. Right now, I need your help with a specific problem (such as potty training). If you are able to help me, I'll be very appreciative. If not, my feelings for and about you won't change." The message received by the child is, "My fate is in the hands of these huge, godlike adults, the undisputed King and Queen of my existence. I had better try my best to do as they ask, or some very bad, never clearly defined things could happen to me. I must be good."

So we set out at this early age in an *attempt to do the impossible: to earn love.* Not only that, but because we desire love all the time, we must be deserving of love continuously. We must be perfect!

There are some positives that come from this mindset. People with this compulsive need to achieve make tremendous efforts at everything they attempt. They can't quit, because defeat is almost like death. If I had a heart attack, a doctor with a poor self-image would be who I'd like treating me. I'd like to go to war with one of these driven people. I know I like them on my side in a game of basketball. They just plain have to win. No other choice exists. What's wrong with winning? The problem isn't with winning. I think winning is great. The problem is that if you *have* to win at everything all the time, the pressure can become unbearable. Losing causes you great pain. Winning brings only a moment of respite until you have to win again.

It's hard for other people to feel real closeness to someone who is constantly trying to be better than they are. This can be a lonely way to live. The accomplishments that you thought (perhaps way down in your subconscious) would bring you love instead cause people to avoid you. Who, no matter how centered, likes to be beaten? It may amaze you to find out that some of the people you "beat" didn't even know there was a contest. It could be they were just out enjoying some activity and having some fun in the doing.

A number of lessons must be learned or the constant pressure and pain of such a life can lead to disaster. Living in this continual state of apprehension can lead to alcohol or drug use to dull the fear and pain. It can lead to cheating in some form, such as in a business situation, with the IRS, or in an attempt to get ahead of the "competition." Such a driven lifestyle can destroy marriages and other relationships. It can also prove very destructive to the individual's health.

The first lesson to learn is that while there may be some question about exactly what love is and how it is attained, you don't achieve it by beating someone. My definition of love is that it is something that is freely given. Love is a verb, a state of being, not a thing that can be purchased, stored, or deserved. You can't earn love. It comes by itself, drawn by love given out. Said another way: If you wish love in your life, give love to others.

Lots of great minds have attempted to give us this message for thousands of years. It is so very hard for some of us to hear because we were conditioned at an early age to believe differently. It's difficult to believe we are so wrong on such a vital issue, and that the answer is so simple. To be loved, we don't have to be perfect, only loving.

Why did our parents condition us to feel we have to deserve their love in the first place? Part of the reason is because their parents probably raised them this way. As a parent of four, I can testify to not having any divine revelations as to how to raise children. I often tell my kids that we're just making the rules up as we go along and trying to do the best we can. (My wife however, claims she *knows*.) Parenthood simply doesn't come complete with an explicit instruction book covering every conceivable situation.

Another reason that some of us were raised in this manner is that our parents loved us very much! They wanted us to succeed. The way to success for them was to never be satisfied, but always try for more.

While historically this hasn't been the path chosen by all cultures and at all times, we were raised in the great Calvinist work ethic. Laziness is the devil's tool! If parents tell their children they loved them, no matter what their behavior, they might get lazy and lay down on the job. Also, most of us wish to be perceived as good parents. Part of being an outstanding parent is to raise children who achieve success. I don't think a lot of thought was given to the curse of living a life where you are never satisfied.

A message we must understand in order to get off this tread mill of earning love is that winning isn't necessary. Now, don't jump out of your comfortable chair. I didn't say that if you are to be happy you can't try or that you must lose. What is necessary is to try your best. Pick a goal that has meaning to you and do your utmost! *The effort*, not the result, is the thing to focus on. Once you have done your best to achieve an accomplishment of worth (for now, let's just say a worthy goal is one that hurts no one else in the achieving and has real meaning in your life), then glory in that good effort, whatever the result. Know that who you are isn't dependent on winning. I don't have any idea of what winning really is anyway. You tell me: Is playing a game that ends with you having a higher score and your opponent hating you, winning? Or would winning be having a lower score, but the affection and admiration of your opponent? If we can't agree on which is winning, is it worth making yourself miserable to pursue victory as a goal?

What ever you decide winning is (I gave up wondering about it years ago), realize it has nothing to do with who you are or your value as a person. We are all blessed with talents and weaknesses in different areas of our lives. Some tasks we can perform effortlessly. Others will be difficult for us no matter how much we practice or how great our effort. Neither winning or losing makes you worthy of love. To connect the results of your actions to who you are is to be sadly and tragically confused. Your life, as was mine, will be filled with "victories" and pain.

"Wait until Vince Lombardi hears this bull." Consider his famous quote: "Winning isn't everything, it's the only thing." And he asked for 11 men that hate to lose—not who love and glory in victory—in order to make a champion. Life isn't a football game. Football lasts a couple of hours. Is that how you choose to live your life; with every play being a fourth down? Few have the strength to sustain this type of effort for long. None can live like this forever.

What I'm trying to tell you is this: You deserve to be loved because you are. Again, it is so simple. Our value is established by the fact we exist. All we need to do for peace in our lives is accept that statement. The contests and constant measuring against each other is simply our crazy idea. No great book I've studied says the one with the most at the end wins. There's even some real debate about what constitutes an end. If some great sage or solon did say such a thing, my question would be the most what? Money? I have a lot, and, in itself, money contains neither peace nor joy. Toys? I doubt many of us accept "toy collecting" as a reason to exist (although our behavior may belie that truth). When you finally got the "car of your dreams," did you feel joy and peace forever? Or did you worry it would be damaged or stolen, or that a friend would get a better one? There are not enough accomplishments or things in this great universe to make a person feel worthy. Having the best office, the perfect crown margins, or the most beautiful home in town will not do it. Feeling worthy is simply a choice we can make.

Others much wiser then I will have to explain the purpose of existence. This is a question that I find fascinating to reflect on, but the scope of the author's talents prevents its discussion here. I can give you a simple answer to another age-old question: How do I get love? If you desire love, simply give it. I've stated it another way to my children as sort of a parable. If you want a back rub, it's easy to attain. Just rub someone else's back. To receive, we first must give.

The Buddhist and Hindu concept of *karma* is simply a spiritual concept of cause and effect. The more love you give, the more will be returned to you. Also, every evil deed and thought will be repaid to you at some time, in some way. St. Paul said, ". . . everyone reaps what he sows." (Galatians 6:7, Revised English Bible) Life gives back to you that which you give out to it. Sow love and reap love. Sow anger or hatred and receive the same. The very good news is that *what you receive in life is yours to control.* What you put into life returns to you. Winning and losing just don't have anything to do with it.

Think for a moment about the people that you admire and enjoy being with. Is it their ruthless drive and selfish wish to achieve that you find so enjoyable? We all can think of a few people that "everyone likes." Try to analyze what makes them so lovable. I believe a large part of the seemingly universal attraction of infants and pets is the fact that they don't judge, but accept. Why is it so hard for us to show the same affection for others seen in any dog, except the mistreated?

"You know, I got this book to help me be a better dentist and perhaps to make more money. Now all I'm reading is a bunch of wishy washy stuff about feelings, values, and such."

OK, Mister Hard-Cold-Facts Dentist. How would you like to experience a day where you did your best, your very best, and no matter what the result was, you were at peace? You know there are things in life you can't control. You let being the best dentist you can be on that given day be enough. You don't insist that all you do be perfection, but do your best possible in every situation. You took joy in that and worked in the peace that such knowledge brings.

More than that, you saw your staff and *every* patient as a being worthy of love, as are you. The kindness that such a mindset creates is noticed and reacted to by everyone who experiences it. Your staff didn't need to be perfect to be respected and complimented. You didn't fear they wouldn't work as hard if you offered some kind words to them.

Remember, my main objective in this book is to show how to produce joy. But ask yourself, at what level of his/her possible performance is this dentist working? Answer: the peak! What do you think his/her stress level is? How do you think his/her staff retention rate would be? How many days a year is this doctor sick? What would be the new patient flow in such an office? More importantly, you have here an individual doing his/her best to help people and feeling good about the very tough job he/she is doing.

This exact type of dentist probably doesn't exist. I'm a Christian, but my goal isn't to be Christ. It's to learn from His life and teachings and to try to come as close as I can to His example. I would suggest it's the same with this loving, relaxed dentist. We have to create a vision of what we're shooting for in the office. We have to clarify our values and then try our best to reach this goal. We can't fail. We just made the goal up; thus it's not possible to hit or miss an imaginary target. No real target exists, except that which our minds have created. All we can possibly do is to strive to get better and better, to become closer and closer to the person we'd like to be. What I'd like to be is a person who helps others and while doing so is filled with joy. What about you?

The way we feel about ourselves flavors every moment of our lives. If we are constantly judging ourselves, we are also prone to judgments of our spouse, children, and staff. It has been my experience that such judgmental behavior is not appreciated. The way to change this unsatisfactory situation is to accept the fact that all of us are created with value. Just accept. Can I prove this to be true? No, I guess not. Can you prove that only by winning can you attain joy? What has your experience been when you have followed this "winning" philosophy? The theory is so easy to test. Go around all day and outperform everyone at everything. Find flaws and errors in others' behavior and point it out to them. Be better than others and win. Now, stop at the end of the day and reap what you just sowed. How do you *feel?* How do others *feel* about you?

I bet you've figured out Part Two of our experiment. Will it kill you to spend one day trying only to do your best (it's the effort, not results that count), to see value in others? To not engage in contests and struggles, but to try instead to give love and affection? Can you force yourself to spend one day in a loving manner? Can we get one hour? Does it scare you that this is so hard and you'll do almost anything but attempt it?

Inside, you already know the answer. It is to love and accept others as your brothers and sisters. My poor explanations of why this is so hard matters little. I know it's tough to act completely loving, even with your loved ones. Please try. Teach yourself that this is the pathway to joy. What can you lose?

Allow me to add a caudal. Despite my beliefs that simply by existing we have worth, I don't believe that all people deserve to have a good self-image. This may seem to contradict all that I have just said, so allow me to explain.

I do believe that we are all of intrinsic value. I also hold that if we pick a *worthy goal* and make an *honest effort* to obtain that goal, we should need nothing else to feel positive about ourselves. Bear in mind the worthy goal and honest effort.

I don't believe that people who manipulate, cheat, and take advantage of others should feel positive about their actions. Their behaviors are their choices, and they are free to change their actions whenever they choose to. As long as their choices are for ends or means that are not worthy, they should feel badly about it. This pain is needed to redirect them to actions that will allow them to find the peace and joy they have as a birthright, but must by their right actions continue to deserve. In Chapter 6 we'll look at pain and attempt to understand that there may be a positive side to this seemingly negative sensation. A dimension in our suffering that can lead to a positive outcome.

Please try my little experiment. Try it at home or at the office. If you spend just a few hours honoring people for their existence, giving love and withholding judgment, I believe it could change your life. It's a tough job we do. Doing it lovingly makes our work and our lives a lot easier and will yield us the joy we desire and deserve.

CHAPTER 5

MORALITY
AND
SELF-IMAGE

I know a lot of people who define morality as doing something without getting caught. A few of my acquaintances of such persuasion aren't even lawyers. But in what manner are morality, self-image, and dentistry interrelated? Even if there is a relationship, why would it interest you? "I want to make money and be successful, not achieve sainthood!" some may be saying.

Please recall a statement we made earlier. In a loose paraphrase, we advised, "Be very careful what you want, for surely you shall get it." It took me 10 years of setting goals and attaining the goals I had set to understand the very real importance of that statement. Only after I had achieved goal after goal and found myself still unfulfilled did I see my error: great effort, wrong goals. I wanted joy and peace, but I worked to attain money.

Chasing after the wrong goals is a little like taking a spelling test, spelling a word correctly, but not spelling the word you were asked to spell. In dental parlance it would be performing a flawless extraction— of the wrong tooth. While what you accomplished is technically correct, nothing of value was achieved. Setting the right goals is the most critical step in the attainment of a rewarding life, yet few want to perform the labor required to be sure the goals they choose are correct for them. They don't want to sit quietly and try to understand who they are and what they believe; they want action! Emerson said, "What is the hardest thing in the world to do? To think for oneself." I completely agree, but he did not say it was impossible.

I taught briefly at the University of Iowa College of Dentistry. I can remember how students making dentures were reluctant to check the extension on their custom trays before starting the impression process. They wanted action! After they had spent four hours, painstakingly border-molding those trays with compound, I'd check their work and frequently find the trays had overextended borders. I'd reduce the compound until I realized the custom tray itself had been too long to begin with. At this point the student had to remove all the lovingly applied compound and begin the process anew.

Are there any parts of your life where you're creating that kind of "action?" I speak of activity without a clearly defined focus and direction. The sort of activity that generates a lot of heat, but little light. Such action would include being busy for the sake of business, without careful thought to what all the business was intended to achieve. If you think you're not guilty of any such behavior, better close the book and reflect a bit. When you are being honest again, we can continue.

OK, so you'll grant me, at least for argument's sake, that for a life to be filled with joy and meaningful achievement, the individual must be working toward a worthy goal. But what is worthy? And how can we tell when we are pursuing such a goal?

Part of the answer to this question lies in the realm of morality. Morality is also inexorably tied to self-image, but let's withhold a discussion of that relationship for the time being.

No goal can be worthy that violates the rights of another. There is no need to quote a great man to prove this point. This is as good a place as any for you to begin to "prove things" using your own experience and your own mind. Reflect back on your life. Remember times when you attempted shortcuts, to get ahead of someone at their expense. Maybe a lie was told, or you cheated on an examination. Perhaps a crown was seated with a margin that deep down you knew you wouldn't place in the mouth of a loved one. Maybe an endo fill was completed, although you knew you were several millimeters short of the desired apical seal.

Think of situations when others took advantage of you. Now, reflect carefully on how all these incidents turned out. When all was said and done, did the person who "took advantage" unfairly really come out ahead?

If you can think of an example where you believe the answer to be *yes*, think more critically. What about the emotional price that was paid internally as a result of the deception? If you concentrate long and hard, you may even begin to see that life is fair! Had I always acted as fairly as I would have liked, that thought would give me comfort. As it is, I'm not certain I want to get what I deserve.

But morality is more closely linked to success than simply not violating the rights of others to advance your self-interests. I heard a tape by Earl Nightingale years ago. He said that if morality or honesty hadn't been invented, they should be, simply as the surest way to assure success.

Another way to express Earl's thought is that honesty is its own reward. These are two seemingly curious statements. How can morality assure success, and in what sense can honesty be its own reward?

Do you deal repeatedly with people you know to be dishonest? Would you continue in a relationship with a business that you knew to be without honor? Even more importantly, isn't trustworthiness one of *the* critical ingredients you look for, in a friend as well as in a business relationship? Aren't such virtues as honesty and fairness what you attempt to teach your children to esteem?

So, what do you think patients expect from you and your office? Do you believe you're so special that you are above these same critical areas of concern in their eyes? If you tell a patient you'll see them at 2 P.M., and you see them at 2:30, what is the impression you've given them concerning your office's trustworthiness? If you quote them a fee, but then change it during treatment, for whatever reason, what is the message they receive? Do they understand that you are a person of honor, willing to sacrifice a short-term gain, to keep a commitment you made? You are judged by your actions much more than your words.

To you parents: "Children more attention pay, to what you do than what you say." If you parents want your kids to have a clean room, the way to achieve it is for you to have a clean home. Your patients and staff as well judge you by your behavior, not mere proclamations. Do you tell your kids to be honest and then cheat on your taxes? Do you ever pocket cash from the office, and then assume none of your staff will embezzle? There exists a word to describe those who say one thing and do another: hypocrite. It is not an epitaph I would choose.

One of the keys to success in dentistry is having a large number of patients who believe in you. These patients are loyal to your office. When you tell them what treatment they need, they believe that you recommend this course of therapy because you care about them and their well-being. They believe the recommendation made isn't for your benefit, but for theirs. This is the result of a bond of trust. Few things are so critical to the success of a dental practice, or any business enterprise, as the existence of an atmosphere of faith.

This same high-trust, low-fear relationship must exist between you and your staff. If it's missing, patients will sense its lack. The true price paid for the last day you and your chairside weren't getting along may have been an extensive and critically needed treatment plan turned down by a patient. The patient may not really understand why he/she said no. Something just didn't feel right. Without trust, patients don't accept treatment, and often they don't return to the office at all. A low-trust environment is not a fun place to be. Would you accept a recommendation and act on it if given by a person you didn't believe in?

Nothing is more important to the acceptance of treatment by patients than their sense of your staff having complete trust in you. It's neat to have FMX and glossy study models. Certainly an intraoral camera to be used in codiagnosis would help in case acceptance. None of it is as critical as this *sensing* by your patient that everyone in the staff trusts, admires, and respects you as a person and as a clinician. You're the guy they would, and do, choose to treat their loved ones.

How is such a relationship achieved? It is *earned* by your respect and trust in them, by codevelopment of goals, by your *unflinching integrity,* and your constant commitment to every patient, not to be perfect, but to be the best you can be. Maybe your patient won't know if a crown's margin is open. What about your hygienist? You can't pay your staff a bonus and receive this critical trust in return. You have to earn it behaviorally. A good friend likes to say, "You can't talk your way out of a problem you behaved yourself into." Think about it.

Yet some dentists squander this trust cheaply. They aren't on time for treatment, clearly showing that:

1. They are too inept to be timely.

2. They don't value the patient or believe their time to be important (as the doctor's time is).

3. Both of the above.

These "sellers of trust" charge a patient to replace a filling done six months before. They make a $65 profit on that day by doing so. They may lose a family of patients or at least forfeit their high regard. Many of that family's friends are told of what they perceive to be dishonorable treatment. The focus in such an office is on the short term. This is because there are no clearly stated long-term goals, or such behavior could never take place. These people don't understand that a reputation for honesty is worth more than gold!

So many books on business stress that "Rule number one, the customer is always right. Rule number two, in case of any questions, refer to rule number one." This is the credo that J.C. Penney built his empire on. Wal-Mart's astonishing growth is based on the same principle. The outstanding book, *In Search of Excellence*, stressed that this is one of the key points emphasized by *successful* businesses worldwide. I don't know if dentists just aren't aware of this incredibly critical ingredient of success, or if in the hubris some doctors fall prey to, feel they are above the rules others must abide by to achieve success. Whatever the reason, our office has been blessed with many new patients who are there because another office "made them wrong."

What type of concrete actions can you take to establish this bond of trust between you and your patient? Once you understand and believe in the concepts, you won't have any trouble finding your own personal answers to that question. When you truly understand and are committed to a value, it takes no effort or willpower to follow that commitment with appropriate actions. You do it because you know it to be right. Internalizing the value, not copying a few tricks, is the critical issue. That said, allow me to give you just a few examples of how my staff and I illustrate this value in our office.

Possibly the best illustration of our true concern and value that we have for our patients is that we make every effort to not keep patients waiting. We'll discuss very carefully how this is accomplished later on and how you must time your procedures exactly to have any hope of running your office in a consistently timely and professional manner. The key ingredient to office promptness is *attitude*. We are a professional group, and as pros we have the skill to work in a timely fashion. This idea, firmly held by each staff member and reinforced continually by me, is the key. No set of rules can take the place of an honest self-image shared by every team member: skilled people do their work on time.

Still, patients do arrive late, emergencies (the real kind, with blood running) do occur, and I (once or twice) have had to retake an impression. When we do fall behind schedule, if it is by a significant amount of time (10 or more minutes behind schedule in our office would be a significant delay), we'll call the next patient and inform them to arrive at our office a little later than they had been scheduled. Sometimes we will do less treatment on a patient, such as doing only two of the three scheduled restorations, to allow us to return to schedule. (We never reduce treatment if by doing so the patient would be required to make an extra office visit. In some cases we have the flexibility to replan our treatment with no delay in the completion of patient care, thus allowing us to get back on track.) Often, the whole staff just pitches in, and with all of us working at a higher level of efficiency, we are soon back on schedule.

Our patients are expected to be on time. If they aren't, we change or reschedule their treatment. (You haven't lost the money, doctor, you'll just earn it later. It's more critical to keep your commitment to the next patient to be on time, and a lot less stressful to everybody. Also, treating late-arriving patients tells them in no uncertain terms that it's not a problem for you if they're late. This isn't the message we wish to communicate.)

On our reception room wall is a sign that states "If you are kept waiting for 10 minutes past your appointment time, please advise our receptionist." Not many people say anything, even the few times we do keep them waiting. I feel the sign is a physical manifestation of our awareness of their value as people. If we are running behind schedule, the patient is told immediately when they arrive, an apology is offered, along with a beverage and a newspaper. When I see them, I'll apologize too and explain what happened. Often the "excuse" is that it was just my fault, and I'm sorry. If a true emergency patient caused the delay, or if a previous patient was late, that is also explained. I doubt the patients we have kept waiting ever fully believe the explanations we offer (except the one where it's all my fault). Of course, we would never tell anything but the complete truth. I do believe they realize our apology and our concern are sincere.

If a patient says it's OK that I kept them waiting, I thank them, but tell them that it isn't alright. Their time is too valuable for us to waste. They may not have a thing to do all day, but I believe everyone feels their time to be important. Not honoring that feeling reflects a disrespect for them as individuals. Such disrespect is undoubtedly the *last* thing you wish perceived by your patients.

Occasionally a filling we have done is lost in the first year or so after it was placed. It doesn't happen often, but when it does I say, "I'm really sorry this restoration has to be replaced. We'll redo it right away, and of course there will be no charge. *We aren't perfect here, but we are honest.*" If a lot of your fillings fail, you need a technique book, a continuing education course, or some time spent observing in another office to figure out the problem. No free restoration makes up for having to retreat the patient.

However, I believe that when a restoration does fail, our solution is as close to making a positive result out of the negative event as is possible. What do you think this does for the bond of trust between you and your patient? Do you think this ever gets mentioned over coffee? How does the person listening to your patient feel when they are charged to have a "new" filling redone by their dentist? Would you like to be perceived as a professional who stands behind his/her work? The worst condemnation I hear from a patient about another dentist is, "He/she cared more about money than he/she cared about me." Please don't let that ever be said about your office.

Allow me to mention one last example of building patient trust out of the many in our office. We quote a fee *in writing* for every procedure treatment planned before the dental work is performed. I personally prefer to know in most situations exactly what financial commitment I'm making before any service is provided. So do our patients. Few people like to be surprised when it comes to pecuniary matters. Our care is expensive, and often a patient is somewhat surprised (read *stunned*) by the estimate. Usually they will think about it for a moment, know the treatment is indicated (thanks to our trust relationship and codiagnosis), and tell us to go ahead. This grateful acceptance of care isn't always the norm when they are told the fee *after* treatment and they no longer have a choice about having the procedure completed.

Let's say you scheduled a DO and while restoring the tooth find mesial caries. We never alter a quoted fee. I tell patients that it's their lucky day and as an early "Christmas present," we're restoring an area of decay we didn't know was there *for no charge*. It may take two minutes more to add that one additional surface to the planned restoration. Isn't the feeling your patient gets about your honesty and commitment to them worth that time? This is one of many examples in our office of value-added services: giving more than was bargained and paid for.

Your other choice in this situation is to tell a person one fee, then bill them at another. If a garage did that to you, would you return your car there for future service needs?

The examples given are a few of many in our office that build high trust patient relationships. Each policy seen by itself means little. What's important is having a whole team of people who understand and are committed to these values. How these values are shown will vary with the individuals in any given office and their unique values. Maybe it's offering a ride home to a patient that came by cab, or loaning an umbrella in a sudden rain storm. Each person on the team will find their own way, special to them, to show their concern. What is important is that the care and values are real. They can't be counterfeited, or you will be seen as the dishonest frauds you are.

Let's return to the topic of self-image. I know we discussed it at length, but no issue is more central to the attainment of joy. As I said previously, I believe some people deserve to have a poor self-image. If your personal values and the subsequent actions that result from these beliefs are self-centered or biased toward advancing your cause at the expense of others, your image of yourself must be consistent with these actions. Any other possibility is self-delusion.

So much has been written on self-image. I guess it reflects the importance of the topic. Let's very quickly peruse what a few experts in the field have had to say on the subject.

In the 1960s Thomas Harris wrote about Transactional Analysis in his book *I'm OK, You're OK*. The idea was to realize you were neat (or OK at least) and sort of talk yourself into believing it. This was a combination of developing self-awareness, then deliberately working to change your beliefs about yourself, thus changing your actions.

Albert Ellis is the creator of the philosophy of Rational Emotive Therapy (RET). This too is a talk-yourself-happy-no-matter-how-you-behave-or-feel concept. Dr. Ellis says that between an event or action and the consequence of that event lies the individual's belief. By being aware of this belief, and changing it, people can control their actions and to some extent their feelings.

An example could be a fender-bender type accident. A person's reaction may be, "This is too awful for words. I'm in big trouble now! How can I be so stupid?" Dr. Ellis suggests that you can change your beliefs to something like, "Well, this is certainly unfortunate, but not unbearable. I'll do what I must to correct this problem. Life will go on, and all will be OK with time." The event, the car accident, is the same. The individual has chosen to change his internal beliefs, and thus the consequences and his feelings about them have changed, too.

I agree with Dr. Ellis to some degree. I think the next time you expose a nerve, or get an angry call or letter from a patient, this type of concept can be of help. We do tend to "awfulize," to quote Dr. Ellis, and make unfortunate situations worse. More importantly, we need to realize that *our reactions are shaped by our thoughts, and we have the ability to control our own thoughts.*

Two key quotes that changed my life:

1. "The beginning of wisdom is the realization that beliefs are choices." I'm sad to say I can't remember who originally said this.

2. "Our life is shaped by our minds. We become what we think about." This is the first line of an ancient Buddhist Scripture book, *The Dhammapada.*

"Beliefs are choices." Things are not inherently good or bad, but we label them so. Killing is bad, unless the person killed threatened the safety and existence of you or your loved ones or if he is an enemy in time of war. In that context, killing can become a virtue. The difference is in what you choose to believe and not the action itself, in this extreme example, the killing of another human being.

A slightly more mundane belief: all people, especially all patients, must like and admire me. Realize that you just made that up. That understanding is the beginning of wisdom. Most of what you suffer over, what you call your "failures" and live in fear and shame of, are simply failures of rules that you created. Outside your own awareness, these values may vary or not even exist. Remember, values have no absolute meaning but exist only in our minds. Despite this, people live in misery or choose to end their lives over made up scenarios of good and bad, right and wrong.

You must see that *our minds* do shape our lives. The best news ever may be that we can control our mind, and by careful study and deliberate choice, we can change what we believe. Said another way, we can realize that joy is a choice. Much of what you believe is an accident of your childhood. It was put in your head before you were mentally able to objectively evaluate the content. It's not good or bad to be Republican or Catholic: usually it's an accident of birth. Similarly, all the rigid rules of conduct you hold yourself to and the anguish you feel when you "fail" to keep them are creations of your mind and not absolute truths.

Most of the pain in your life is *self-inflicted*, and for it to stop, only your mindset needs to be altered. You have no obligation to perfection, only to trying your best. The way this change comes about is through a deliberate and searching examination of your most deeply held values. Carefully evaluate all the things you always knew to be true. Do you truly believe in them, or did someone just tell you that you should?

I tell my kids that any question that can't be answered by looking in a mirror (i.e., by self-reflection) isn't worth answering. Not only that, but by wasting time concerning yourself with things beyond your control, you are distracted from the truly important things in life, the value issues where you can have control. Yet most of us spend our time and energy bemoaning the *outside* world and struggling to change that, be it patients, staff, or family.

Recall the riots in Los Angeles over the Rodney King verdict. The eternal cry is for government to step in. (And hasn't government intervention worked so well for us in the past!) The universal cry is for "other people" to change and behave in a manner more consistent with our perception of "proper behavior." Few are saying that I must change my individual feelings about race, or that each of us must examine what we feel to be right in dealing with others.

I can't change what has happened in L.A. I can make friends with a black girl in a girls' home in our town, and I can write to a black lady prisoner in a Florida jail. (I was involved in both activities before the tragedy in L.A., yet these remain valid examples of individual action that can make a difference.) You can change the world with your actions. I believe only individual efforts are effective anyway, despite our tendency to wait for the proper people to "do something" to solve problems for us. This premise of personal responsibility is as valid concerning the totality of the world we live in as it is for the "little world" of our dental offices.

The reason we look so hard outwardly for answers is that we are so frightened to look inside. Let me give you permission to take that look inward. Find the truly wonderful person who lives there. Become his/her friend and try to understand what he/she believes in and who he/she would really like to be. Take this understanding and work to become on the outside a person whom this "inside you" would admire. Socrates is supposed to have said that the greatest way to live with honor is to become what we pretend to be. All value clarification consists of is the discovery of what you believe and changing your behavior to become consistent with that view.

Such a change, though it takes time and effort, is the only answer to finding joy. Happiness is a state of mind. It exists nowhere but inside you. Looking anywhere else simply avoids the truth.

Let's study a few quotes from great minds of different nations and times as they relate to our topic:

Solomon (in Proverbs 23:7): "As he thinketh in his heart, so is he." (King James Version)

Wayne Dyer, in *You'll See It When You Believe It*, shares the following quotes:

> Spinoza: "I saw all things I feared, and which feared me, had nothing good or bad in them save insofar as the mind was affected by them."

> Abraham Lincoln: "People are about as happy as they make up their minds to be."

> Shakespeare: "There is nothing either good or bad, but thinking makes it so."

Such a search and discovery as we have just described will make your life joyful. It will not make your life free of pain. Pain is your ally and friend. To deny or attempt to wish pain away is to choose to no longer grow. Let's now examine the issue of pain and the part it plays in our lives. Is it possible for pain to be our friend and ally?

CHAPTER 6

◆

CAN PAIN
BE OUR FRIEND?

I've admitted earlier that I find dentistry to be hard work. Some days in the office seem composed of irritation, agitation, and apprehension, roughly in equal parts. Taken together, these feelings = pain. Unfortunately, when I leave my office after such a day, guess what I bring home to share with my family? The stray AIDS virus is left at the office for the laundry people to worry about, but it takes more than OSHA to make a dentist leave an upsetting day there, too. I submit that pain is also a contagious disease, often shared with those innocents closest to us.

Can this pain be our friend? A strange question, you say? Allow me to ask another. Do you know anyone living whose life is free of pain? I think we can say that pain is a ubiquitous part of the human condition, more so even than dental disease. If we agree that we can't avoid pain, then how can we best deal with it? The answer of the masters over the ages: *accept it.*

I have read and studied many sources in my efforts to understand. The ancient Hindu saying "There is but one God or Truth; the sages call

Him by many names" seems true to me. If the writings and ideas we discuss here wander from nation to nation and philosophy to philosophy, please accept it as evidence of how diligent my search has been. To me, it's exciting to see the same ideas in ancient Greek, Hindu, Buddhist, Christian, and modern psychological thought. The same concepts repeated throughout the ages, races, and cultures indicates to me a ring of truth contained in the message, even if the sages have called this truth by many and varied names.

That was a long explanation to introduce one short statement. This is the first of Buddha's Four Noble Truths, which comprise the core of his teachings. The first truth and the topic we'll deal with here is this: "Life Is Pain."

The key to living happily and growing as a person is accepting the fact that all have pain in life. It is both a natural and necessary part of our lives. Don't waste energy and time trying to avoid pain. Such a thing isn't possible. We learn to accept pain when we understand what it is: simply a signal that change is needed. Such a message should generate no fear in us once it is accurately perceived.

The idea that if we are in pain, something is wrong (maybe even *we* are wrong) only adds guilt to the pain that already exists. Also, the behavior that we adopt in our attempt to avoid the legitimate pain needed to guide us to changing behavior, such as drinking, taking drugs, abusing food or people, only leads to greater pain at a later date. Sadly, these destructive distractions also allow us to delay implementing the needed changes in our life that the pain was signaling and thus delays our growth.

Let's start easily. What is the meaning or purpose of pain when you put your hand on a hot coal? Is it not that a "change" is needed? The change required here is a simple, physical one: move your hand! When the proper change is made, the painful message stops. Why do you believe that the pain caused by emotion is any different? Turmoil inside of us is also a signal of change needed. This change can be of two types:

1. A change in behavior, because our current behavior is in violation of our beliefs. There are dentists who leave decay under fillings. I see their work. I hope and pray for everyone's sake that the knowledge of this causes them pain and will lead to a change in their behavior.

2. A change in our beliefs, because what we believe isn't an accurate reflection of reality (such as a belief that everything we do must turn out perfectly, or we are failures). To remain sane in dentistry, we must stop demanding perfection, both of ourselves and our fellow practitioners. The best of us will miss an area of decay occasionally, even when we are giving our best effort at that moment. I tell patients that's why God gave us 32 teeth. One mistake in dentistry rarely kills anyone. (If a brain surgeon happens to read this, please take this opinion advisedly.)

Let's quickly summarize our points: Accept pain by understanding that it is a harbinger of our need to change. What we must change is our behavior or our beliefs. While change is often unpleasant, it is only by change that we can grow. It's been said that everyone wants to grow; no one wants to change. It would be nice if that were possible, but in this world growth must be accompanied by that unpleasant, scary entity, change.

Many of us attempt to hide from pain. We deny we have pain, use drugs to make its symptoms go away, or distract our brains with compulsive activity (maybe if we aren't still, we won't have to think). This activity can be anything from being a workaholic, to jogging, to doing church work, to having an affair. The point is the same: to hide us from our pain and the condemnation of our own thoughts. Perhaps worse than the pain itself are the feelings of shame at our lack of perfection that has caused the pain in the first place. We all know that doctors and the first-born kids should be perfect!

But I speak of the past. Now we know that our beliefs are choices. We know that we have the power to examine our values and change them if we feel that to be best. We can now greet pain as we would a smoke alarm. Certainly not a pleasant thing, all noise and light, but designed that way to surely get our attention and give us a much-needed message. Both pain and the fire alarm have the ability to save our lives.

I remember an old Cheech and Chong joke from the 1970s. "Pain, much as fear, is just God's way of punishing us." It never struck me as funny, just frightening. Now I believe it contains more truth than poetry. Pain has a purpose, which is to "punish us" (or create unpleasant ·feelings), to show us that a new path is needed. Not God, but our own behavior leads to the need, or lack of the same, for the message of pain in our life. "As you sow, so shall you reap." "What goes around, comes around." "You get out of life what you put into it." Are you beginning to see that people have tried to tell you this before?

Let me give you an example in my own life of pain, the messenger. As I mentioned, I currently see patients about 100 days a year. That is my *choice*, arrived at finally only through the assistance of a lot of pain. When I worked a more normal 200-plus days a year, my blood pressure and weight were up, my energy and ability to sleep were down. I was committed in my life to hard work and obtaining money. Those were the tokens that I chose to use to keep score in my life.

My dad had a big influence on my thoughts in this arena. Once started in a manic, success-at-all-costs direction, society rewards this path with good grades, financial remunerations, and the praise of your peers. It's also very easy to find books and continuing education classes to help you refine this quest of becoming a perfect working machine.

Certainly hard work and achievement in and of themselves aren't wrong. But I couldn't sleep well, was no fun to be with, and generally blamed everyone else for my misery. I'd tell my poor family, the ones I had no time for, that I was doing it all for them. I can't remember that they had ever asked me to. Of course, I also blamed them for much of my unhappiness. If I ever thought that maybe I was the one mistaken, I had only to check my material achievements to reassure myself that indeed, all my distress was caused by others. I had proof, in the bank, that I was right.

Nothing is caused by others! To think so gives these others control of you. If you are unhappy with anything in your life, *you can change it.* That's the good news, that you can change anything in your life you are unhappy with. Here's the bad: *you* have to do the changing. A scary thought for most. It's not your patients, staff, family, or friends' duty to make you happy. Nothing good can occur until you are willing to accept complete responsibility, not just for your actions, but for your feelings. Happiness is something inside.

But, what if I'm bed-ridden, sick, and dying? What if I lose my job, or a friend or loved one is sick? That surely isn't my fault or responsibility. Who could be happy under such awful conditions? Those who choose to be! All people living with any of the situations we've just described have the same physical problems. The reality of their situation we assume can't be changed. But the attitude of the individual is still theirs to control. They can choose to be angry and bitter at life. That is their right. They can also choose to accept what can't be changed. Some may even look for a reason or blessing in their misfortune and go on to deal with the reality of their existence in a positive way, using their experience to grow. Thousands of stories exist about people who have overcome devastating tragedies to become successful. The reason these stories are so loved and treasured (*Rocky* is a recent, if trite example) is that each of us deep down knows the potential for such triumph exists in us too.

Do you deal with the reality of your existence in a positive way and use it to grow? When life hands you a lemon, as surely it will to all of us, do you consciously look for the ways to turn that lemon into lemonade?

Back to my misery. It got so bad that I was forced to take at least some responsibility in an attempt to fix the mess all the other people had gotten me into. My pain was so pervasive that it forced me to even question the main values of my life. Was hard work, money, and the admiration of others what existence was all about?

Here's where I caught a huge break! I was so dogged in the pursuit of what I saw as my desires, that before I wore my body and mind out completely, I had achieved what I thought I wanted. I had a million dollars in the bank, no debt, a very successful practice, and the appreciation of people whose opinion had meaning to me. Having already achieved all my goals, I could be certain that my unhappiness wasn't caused by frustrated ambitions. What remained was an awareness that my distress came despite achieving all that I had desired.

I was very lucky because had my body given out sooner, I doubt I would have ever questioned my own values. I would undoubtedly have blamed my unhappiness on my inability to achieve my goals. Some of you may not have achieved your goals yet, but have attained my misery. I hope that this message will help you to see the light before you reach the level of unhappiness I sunk to. If it doesn't, at least when you get to your emotional bottom (and actively seek new answers to life's questions), maybe you'll be able to use this information as a rope to help pull you back up.

So, good effort, wrong goals! Forty years of my life, focused in the wrong direction. It reminds me of the story of the not-too-bright deer hunters, who were lucky enough to shoot a big buck. They were dragging him feet first to the car, but the huge rack of antlers kept catching in the brush. Another hunter saw them, and suggested they pull the deer by the horns instead of by the feet. They tried this approach, and one hunter said, "That guy was right. We're sure making a lot better time this way." "Yes," the other hunter agreed, "but we keep getting further from the car."

So how could I turn my "deer" around? My feelings were the keys. I started by accepting responsibility for how I felt and behaved (and gave up all the fun of blaming others). I began to do more of what I liked and less of what I didn't. In other words, my behavior changed as I grew more in touch with my emotions. Most importantly, I needed to clarify my values. I didn't really believe money to be the solution to life's problems, that is just what I had been taught. My dad never had much money. For him, money may have seemed the answer, but I doubt it really is for anyone. All I knew was I had lots of it, and it sure wasn't solving life's problems for me. A lot of deep thought and awareness of my true feelings helped me to begin to identify the things I held in true esteem. The question I asked over and over was, Did that activity, event, or person make me feel happy? Slowly, my values began to be clearer to me.

Armed with this new awareness of what I truly valued, I set out to state my own personal beliefs. I won't bore you with my new beliefs. They are scattered throughout these writings if you are curious. They have no meaning to you for two reasons:

1. They are always changing. As I continue to grow and evaluate my feelings, my beliefs continue to evolve. Emerson said in *Self Reliance*, "A foolish consistency is the hobgoblin of little minds." To be consistent is not to grow.

2. They are my beliefs. They have nothing to do with you. They aren't right or wrong. If you don't comprehend this, you better go back to the beginning of the book, or at least think long and hard on this point.

Stephen R. Covey has written a marvelous book entitled *The 7 Habits of Highly Effective People*. I would like to share with you one thought from his writings. I hope your readiness to understand and my ability to explain can make it clear. Mr. Covey states that *proactive people subordinate feelings to values*. The opposite of this (i.e., placing your feelings of the moment before your values), yields depression.

Proactive people are those who understand that *they* control their lives. These wise individuals base their behavior on what they believe and value, not on their feelings. They will forgo pleasure of the moment to do the right thing. Maybe they choose not to drink (as I now do) because they know the pleasant feeling is ephemeral and takes away from reality. Maybe they choose to be honest, even when it is more comfortable to not tell the truth, because they understand that suffering the short-term discomfort of a painful truth is easier than living with the problems caused by long-term deceit.

To live for the pleasure of the moment leads to depression. I know of no happy drunks or drug users. They eventually become "recovering" or dead. Do you really get joy from the subtle lies you tell? Living in a house you haven't paid for, driving a car you can't afford, wearing clothes to indicate a status you haven't achieved? Is this true joy? Do the people who see you admire and respect you, or do they envy and avoid you? Do you like phonies? Do you make real friends based on lies? How about long-term patient commitments based on using patients for your gain? Who is fooled, and who gains an advantage?

Here is what you must know. These behaviors are sad attempts to fool people into thinking you are all right. You feel miserable in the deception. The debt gets in bed with you when you try to sleep. It is between you and your wife at the most intimate moments. It colors honest relationships with people who could be your true friends. It all leads not to joy, but to pain.

Saddest of all, even if this grand scheme worked and everyone was fooled into believing you are wonderful, the only person who really matters would know the truth. You yourself won't be fooled by these "delusions of adequacy."

The answer to this painful dilemma lies in a reassessment of your values. Come to see that who you are really is all right. You always were and always will be. Nothing you can do will change that fact. You simply need to acquire the clarity to see it, and all the pretense will drop away. All your need for material accouterments will be like a winter coat in summer, abandoned because it no longer has a purpose. Tremendous energy is now freed for the things of true value to you. Maybe it's growing closer to your family, staff, and friends. Maybe it's to learn to really care about the patients who trust you. The energy will allow you to become the best dentist you can be. You may even accept yourself as you are, a less-than-perfect person, doing a hard job to the best of his abilities, and *blessed* with the opportunity to make a positive difference in the life of others.

If you understand this, the rest of the book will be easy to grasp. It's simply a lot of tips to help you serve others more efficiently, in our case, through the venue of dentistry. Because you serve well, you will be rewarded in whatever way you choose. *If you give the service, you can't escape being rewarded.* In case you choose money as part of the reward, we'll spend some time on how to make it and save it. I think you'll find, with the right philosophy, that making and keeping money is very easy. I suspect some of you have already discovered that without the right philosophy, it's virtually impossible.

Let me complete my own story (I don't want to leave myself in misery). I now choose to work eight days a month and will cut back to six days soon. I felt guilty for a long time because I worked so little. People tried in many ways to point out that working so little was wrong. I realized that for me, the frantic search for material wealth was a learned reflex, not a clearly thought-out decision. I believe I felt that money would prove me to be all right as a person and give me security.

I learned I already was all right, so reason number one disappeared. Megan's head injury taught me much about security. Namely, that no "thing" can provide it. Objects such as money, cars, and toys are lifeless. I put my stock today in living things such as feelings, ideas, and people.

People ask me, "What do you do with your time?" I tell them the truth, anything I want to. Said another way, what brings me bliss. I know some of you want me to tell you what brings joy. Stop a minute and think how sad such a request is. It indicates a tremendous detachment from your own feelings. If you had this thought, stop and reflect long and hard. The message of this book is that you don't need this book or anything else. You simply need to reattach to who you are and begin a wonderful journey of rediscovery. The ticket for this journey is your feelings.

I recorded my life's journey, actually wrote down what I remembered from different periods of my life. Try it for yourself. Try to recall some things that happened before the age of five. Rediscover that wonderful child. Know that he or she still exists in you. The harder it is for you to recall, the more your emotions are blocked, the more you *need* to make the effort. Try it for just a few minutes a day if you can stand no more. This effort too will get easier.

Let's briefly sum up the information to date:

1. Get in touch with your feelings. Lose your fear of emotions, even of pain. These feelings are simply a part of you.

2. Use these feelings to help clarify your values. This process will take a lifetime, as long as you continue to grow. It never becomes boring. It also isn't scary when you realize that you can't be right or wrong. It's the searching process itself that is important, not the result.

3. Based on these clear values, goals that *accurately* reflect your true beliefs can be set. I used to set goals and work to achieve them. That in itself isn't enough if you wish happiness as a result of your labors. Without clarified values, goals may do more harm than good. Don't be guilty of dragging your deer away from the car, no matter how fast you can go.

4. Remember that man has the ability to control his own thoughts and thus, to some extent, how he feels. Within the context of clear values and proactive goals, the ability to control is good. Without clear and appropriate goals, it often is used for self-delusion and so arrests growth.

The rest of this book can be seen most productively as a guide to show you how to implement this philosophy in the context of a highly successful dental practice. This is my definition of highly successful: one that allows us to give the maximum amount of service to our patients while having fun and growing both as individuals and as members of a team.

As you read on, hold every idea you consider emulating up to this criteria: will implementation of this idea bring me closer to my clear goals? Will it help me to better serve, to grow, or to have more joy?

A SHORT ESSAY ON GOALS, GOAL SETTING, AND VALUES

I have mentioned goals throughout the course of this book. I believe it only proper that I share with you what expertise I may have in the areas of goal setting and achieving. Yet I do so with very mixed emotions, because I personally no longer think goals are an important or even a positive influence on my life journey. The duties once assigned to goals in my life have been superseded by a focus on values.

Values are subjects which require a great deal more clarification, time, thought, and effort than do goals to be effective adjuncts in your quest to achieve. Due to the difficulty inherent in the value clarification and self-discovery process, it may be that proper goal setting is a vital early step to achievement on the path to a value oriented existence.

Please remember that all goals are targets that you create. *They are nothing more than fabrications: things you made up! Don't ever be guilty of the egregious fault of sacrificing a value to achieve a goal.* Let me give you an example of the potential danger inherent in selecting goal completion over values.

Let's assume you set a goal for a certain level of production per day in your office. If you recommend care for patients that you would not have suggested before setting your goal, or perform work below your true standards to achieve this goal, how do you believe such behavior will affect you emotionally? The great danger inherent in the pursuit of goals is to lose track of your beliefs in their mindless pursuit.

I hope this warning will suffice. I feel something akin to my emotional state when I've handed a gun to one of my children for the first time. Guns can be tools of great usefulness in some situations (I get few quail without one), but it also contains the possibility of great misfortune if improperly used.

There is a story I have heard many times that establishes the efficacy of goal setting. It concerns a study completed at an Ivy League school. On the day of graduation it was found something like 4% of the class had *written goals* (in truth there are no other kind, as we'll see). The same class was studied 30 years later. Only the 4% with written goals were financially independent. As I said, I've read this story several times. I accept it to establish a principle, but things so neatly wrapped and tied to make a point are seldom fact.

Despite my incredulities concerning the veracity of this epic, there is no question in my mind that goal setting does work. I used the technique for years with great "success" (i.e., I got what I thought I wanted).

How then to approach this mythical beast, *goals?* To exist a goal must meet certain criteria. These include:

1. A written statement of the situation you wish to deal with as it now exists. This must be very detailed and specific.

2. A written statement of the precisely desired outcome you'd like from your efforts (your goal).

3. The goal must be stated in very specific terms, including a date by which you will have accomplished it.

4. If at all humanly possible, there must be a way to measure your progress on the road to attainment.

5. You must devise a method by which you will chart and monitor this progress and create a plan to allow you to adjust your efforts if you find you're not on course to reach your objective.

6. After the attainment of your goal (we do attain that which we truly desire), a system to reset and monitor our future efforts and progress should be in place.

Let's look at a couple of examples to clarify these concepts:

1. My weight is currently (list the date) 177 pounds.

2. I wish my weight to be 155 pounds.

3. I would like to achieve this goal by the end of a 90-day period. (Goal is clear and very specific.)

4. I will place a chart by the bathroom scales and record my weight on the chart in writing every Monday morning.

5. I plan on reducing my caloric intake to 1,500 calories per day and exercising aerobically at least 30 minutes per day. I will join the fitness class at the YMCA today.

6. Once my goal weight of 155 is attained, I will continue to write my weight down on the bathroom chart and also continue at least three exercise events of a minimum duration of 30 minutes per week.

That's a very simple, straightforward example of goal setting. Let's run through the system again and use a dental situation for an example:

1. Our current average office production (include the date) for the last 12-month period was $20,000 per month.

2. I wish to increase that production to $30,000 per month.

3. I would like to achieve this average monthly production by the end of the next 12-month period.

4. We will calculate the average daily production needed in our office. (Divide days worked per month into $30,000, i.e., 15 days worked means we must produce $2,000 per day) to achieve this goal.

5. This figure will be recorded on the top of each daily schedule along with the scheduled production for that day. In addition, a running total for the month to date, plus or minus our goal, will be displayed. Our progress will be discussed at our regular staff meetings, and our plans to attain this goal adjusted as indicated by our progress. Our current plans to achieve our goal include:

   a. Begin to time all procedures we perform to allow scheduling for maximum production (covered in Chapter 12).

   b. Increase our emphasis on treatment planning of quality care (read crown and bridge).

   c. Become more adept at financial arrangements so our patients can afford this needed treatment. Look into credit cards, dental charge cards, and an in-office hookup to a credit company to allow us to more accurately evaluate the patient's financial condition. (We currently use all three of these entities in our office.)

6. Once our goal is achieved, we will continue to post our production numbers in the above-detailed manner, as well as consider taking courses on orthodontics, veneers, cosmetic care, and implants to further increase our productive capabilities. (My dad always said, "If you're going to be a bear, might as well be a grizzly!") So let's take *all* the courses.

I used to have written goals kept at both my office and my home for the following six facets of my life.

   1. Professional

   2. Personal

3. Financial (my favorite)

4. Family and friends (social)

5. Spiritual

6. Physical (I was always going to lose weight and exercise more.)

I would be actively working on only two of these goals at any one time. To attempt to achieve them all concurrently, leads to total frustration (if not a breakdown or heart attack). I always had the two goals I was actively engaged in achieving openly displayed, such as taped to my bathroom mirror, so I saw them each morning and night, or displayed prominently on my desk at the office.

I can recommend two excellent books that deal with goals (as well as a host of other valuable, enjoyable, and interesting things).

See You at the Top, by motivational author and lecturer Zig Ziglar. (A super guy to listen to, and this book contains the best and most concise explanation of goals I have ever read, and I've studied plenty.)

Franklin the Autobiography, Author unknown (You do get that joke, don't you? It's all about Ben.)

I may question the benefits of goal setting today. I do not question the need for a clear focus if you wish to achieve in any endeavor. Goals can give you this focus. In the hands and minds of those serious about success (you lazy folks are safe), they are indeed powerful tools.

Allow me one more attempt at moralizing. Think of goals as weapons. Use the processes of value clarification and self-discovery. This is how you aim the gun. As with any weapon of power, you must be absolutely sure of your direction of focus before you pull the trigger.

The proper setting of goals and the required following through can attain for you whatever you desire. Of course, you must still do the work required to attain the object you desire. Just be sure this rocket isn't pointed at you before you touch it off.

CREATING
EXCELLENCE
IN A
DENTAL TEAM

CHAPTER 7

COMMUNICATION
AND
TEAM BUILDING

In this chapter we'll turn all of our internal efforts, the steps of self-discovery and personal evaluation we've been so involved with to this point in an outward direction. Through the communication systems that this chapter will cover in great detail, our clarified values and goals will be transmitted to our staff. The net result of this process is the creation of a true team of people, where before there had existed only a collection of individuals who happened to work under one roof.

A team is a group of people working together toward the attainment of a worthy goal. As we have discussed, I'm sure a book could and likely has been written as to what a "worthy" goal is. For this discussion's sake, let's define it as attempting the achievement of a task consistent with our carefully thought-out values. This achievement must be attained without taking advantage of another.

Your team will develop goals together as a part of the team-building process that begins with internalizing the information contained in the following chapters.

A major goal of mine in the early years of my professional existence was simply developing the team itself. Once this is accomplished, I believe you'll find both the setting and achieving of worthy goals an easy task to complete. Tremendous creative energy is released by a group of individuals with one will, directed by both an inspired leader (you) and a clearly defined mission statement. I can promise you an exciting journey ahead.

A great deal of this book is devoted to communication and team building. Why bother? You're the boss, and you don't need someone to hold your hand on life's journey, do you? What's wrong with giving your staff orders, and if those orders aren't followed, you fire those people and hire new ones? (I believe making staff walk the plank for disobedience is no longer either popular or legal, and it's rather impractical if you practice in land-bound area.)

Allow me to answer the above query (as I am wont to do) by asking some further questions in order to stimulate your ability to self-discover the best possible answer for your situation. Do you ever feel lonely in your office? Have you ever said (perhaps to your spouse), "It's always all of 'them' against me?" What would it be worth to have not only physical, but emotional support from your staff every day? The work we do is so difficult. Some patients and procedures make it almost impossible at times. Can you imagine working with a group of friends? People who share and understand your dreams and goals, who are there to support you, just as you are there to support them? None of us is an island, and no wise man would choose to stand alone. Our problem in the past was that we never knew how to get everyone to work together. I can't imagine that any dentists enjoy practicing in a state of isolation from their co-workers. What we suffered from was "a failure to communicate."

The proper medication for the previously named malady is an office communication system, a method whereby you can accurately share the values and goals you have created with your staff. You will become a true office leader, because you now have a destination to lead to: the land of your vision, created by the process we have already discussed. With the systems we'll now unveil, this vision can be shared effectively with the people you spend so much time with and that impact on your success and happiness so greatly: your staff.

Let's begin by describing the task of a leader. Many of you, by your actions if not your thoughts, consider a leader as someone who gets to be boss and tell others what to do (if not where to go). This type of leadership is similar to moving a rope by pushing it. Consider the concept for a minute. No one will argue that pushing a rope will move it. The problem lies in control and efficiency of motion.

A true leader is in front, pulling the rope, not behind pushing. The way we get in front as a leader is to:

1. *Create a clear vision* of where your leadership is headed.

2. *Share this vision* with the people around you to give them a sense of direction and to inspire them.

3. Continue to *articulate this vision* at every possible opportunity. Never fall prey to the fallacy that "I've already told them what I believe." Do you believe that you can tell your spouse and children that you love them once, and then never need to mention it again? Find every way you can to illustrate the goals and values that you esteem, and *never stop.*

I would caution you on one point. I think the greater the variety of ways you find to express your vision, the better. Different people will receive understanding and motivation from varied approaches, and fresh and inspiring presentations of your vision will add new energy to your dreams. However, don't ever sacrifice the clarity of your vision for variety. Don't use analogies that make your feelings less clear just to say things in a different way.

I've frequently described the communication program that exists in our office to other professionals. Be assured, the development of this system is not inexpensive, either in time, effort required, or money. The response I often hear is: "I can't afford to take the time that a concept like that will require." Can you afford the loneliness that comes from no one understanding? How much does it cost you to continually have conflict with a staff member (in gut lining, as well as lost efficiency and joy)? What expense is involved when you realize you must fire a member of your staff? I've heard it said many times that to hire and to train a new staff member costs $10,000. While I can't prove that figure true, what is the expense of doing a second molar crown prep with your brand new chairside assisting?

I hope these examples help put the time and price of an office team-building and communication system in a different perspective.

With a little thought to your own experience, I'm sure you can add a few more dollars as well as frustrations to this total (maybe lost production, decreased collections, messed up insurance—see what I mean?) I think the potential pitfalls we've just discussed more than justify any expenses occurred in team building, but as a way to ascertain the true value of a communication system, this negative measure of reduced loss doesn't even scratch the surface.

The spirit and creative potential that is generated by a true dental team has to be experienced to be believed. Once a true team has been created, the positive effect of the growth of your practice, the joy of working together as a unit, the accelerated flow of new patients attracted by the atmosphere created, and the added productive capability will make all other considerations seem minuscule in comparison.

The series of steps that is our communication system includes three distinct parts:

1. A daily staff meeting and "clearing"

2. A structured communication exercise that all staff must participate in during our two-hour, biweekly staff meetings

3. Individual consultations with each staff member, held once per quarter

Each of these steps is essential to our office's growth and well-being. They were developed separately and slowly in our office, and each has value in its own right. It took me years to realize that when combined with a philosophy of practice (physically embodied in our purpose), the three steps of our communication system had a synergistic quality that multiplied their effectiveness when all are performed together.

STEP 1. Morning staff meeting and clearing. We have a pretty busy practice. A lot of days I will personally see 40 patients (including hygiene checks). I feel it is essential for me to really *know* each and every one of these people it is my privilege to care for. We have over 5,000 active patients, and my memory's not that good.

I realize a lot of you won't like to hear this, but I get to my office by 6:30 each morning to prepare for our 7:30 staff meeting. I review the file of each patient I'm to see that day. I personally make decisions on what X-rays each may need and note it on the schedule. I don't think as doctors we should create and blindly follow generic rules concerning patient treatment for our convenience at the expense of our clients. I mean rules like how often to take X-rays on each patient. Do you really believe a patient who is totally free of any history of dental disease needs the same films as a geriatric patient with active root caries? The frequency and the type of films needed are decisions I make for all patients, based on their own unique dental histories.

Another subject I review on each patient's record is consistency in treatment recommendations. Do you ever recommend home care such as a fluoride rinse and not follow that recommendation up during each office visit with staff reinforcement? Who goes through and makes sure all previously diagnosed treatment has been completed? (Or does no one else preauthorize treatment and then find at the next recare appointment that it's never been performed?) How do we look when we tell a patient that a crown is needed on one visit, and never mention it again? Do you think the patient doesn't remember? What do you think they believe about our office and how important the care we suggest is? How seriously do you believe they will take our further recommendations, assuming they stay in the practice? (I wonder if I could write a whole book of nothing but questions?) Consider all these examples as they pertain to your desires to develop a high-trust office.

Are you ever frustrated when all the materials you'll need for a procedure aren't set out in advance? With the complexity of new materials and types of treatment available today, a complete set-up would be difficult to achieve in some situations, even if your assistant were able to read your mind (a scary thought!). Moments lost when we have to stop treatment to find a needed material or instrument do not add meaning to my life. Even experienced staff appreciate a written reminder clearly noted on the daily schedule of the exact materials we'll need on difficult or unusual cases. For example, will the post buildup you're performing at 10 A.M. require Tenure, Fuji II, a Dentatus Post, or some combination of the above?

Almost every day we will experience changes in our patient schedule due to failures or late cancellations. I briefly review the proposed treatment plans for each of our patients scheduled to be seen that day. Since they will already be coming to the office, a change in the planned sequence of their care may be the best and easiest way to fill openings in our schedule. Instead of the two restorations we had planned to do that day, we switch plans to a crown we already have planned, and our schedule is once again filled. Our patient isn't inconvenienced and our staff doesn't have to frantically scramble trying to find someone available on short notice (who usually arrives 20 minutes late anyway). Over the years a lot of hours of productive treatment time has been salvaged in this manner. Since I only see patients eight days a month, I do like to be productive on my rare office guest appearances!

All these critical items, and many more, I note in writing on each day's schedule. At 7:30 *all the staff are present.* (Did you notice that I said at 7:30 all our staff are present? Are all your staff on time—always?)

One person late for a staff meeting is an annoying way for me to begin the day. In the past, when a staff person was tardy, I used to "talk" to them, threaten them, pout—you get the picture.

Then a moment of genius! In our office, if you punch in *one minute* or more late, you are fined $2. The money goes into a "kitty" used to purchase the entire staff's food of choice (our choice runs strong to donuts).

Today it takes us quite a few weeks to raise enough "Late Fees" for even a dozen donuts. We have become an unusually prompt group of individuals. Who enforces this rule? The whole donut-eating bunch of us, working as a team. (Promptness is a value we all support.) Late and chagrined staff members are now greeted with grateful applause and seen as what they truly are: the bearer of future food! We now *have fun* with what was once a major annoyance that threatened to start our day off in a negative vein.)

When everyone is present, I lead a discussion concerning that day's proposed treatment for each patient. Every member of our staff may have some input. The front office may add that a particular patient is having a problem with finances. "Please don't do any unscheduled treatment without checking with us." Hygiene may want us to check flossing, how a mechanical brush is working, or whether more fluoride or Peridex is needed. Some kind soul may remind me of a divorce, an upcoming wedding, a recent vacation, or a loss in the family (and thus reduce for me, at least for the moment, the taste of my own shoe leather). All this information can be exchanged concerning our entire daily schedule, including hygiene, in about 10 minutes.

Do you think this information adds to our production for the day? What does it tell my staff about *my commitment* to our office and to our patients? How do you feel when the M.D. you've seen for years obviously can't remember who you are? How do you think our increased efficiency due to this preparation changes the perception of us in our patient's eyes? Are we seen as caring about them as individuals, and not just seeing them as a set of teeth with an attached wallet?

This review of all patients and their proposed treatments is critical, but it's after this is completed that we get to the essential part of our morning meeting: the "clearing." This involves everyone taking about a minute and sort of reading to the rest of us their own current emotional barometer. Maybe today the news they share is about something neat that has happened in their lives. That's great! After they share this good news with our team, we can all celebrate.

But consider this scenario: all morning long, your chairside is distant and distracted. She fumbles and stumbles. You bite your tongue, until it goes too far. Then you set her straight, and how!

Do you think it would have made a difference in your feelings toward her, and how the day went, if in a morning clearing session, she had shared with you that she had just suffered the loss of a loved one? Maybe it's a sick child or a family member in the hospital that has caused her distraction. Maybe she's sick but so loyal to you that she's doing her best to get through the day. Would that knowledge change your perception of reality? I'll leave it to you to put a value on such information.

My perception of the greatest value to come from our clearing is this: a demonstration that we all care for and support each other, both as individuals and team members. Maybe today will be a day when you're not at your best. How would it feel to be surrounded by a group of friends who understand and care? Friends who will be there to support you just as you've been there in support of them? What will be the difference in your patient's perception of the team that day? Will they see dissension or mutual care and support? If you were a patient, which atmosphere would you favor?

An additional benefit of this brief time we spend together is the chance all of us get to know each other as people (and not just fellow workers) a little better. Before patients arrive and our commitment to their care correctly overshadows our personal concerns, we have this time to be just friends and share the good and bad that life brings us all.

Often a staff person's only comment is "I'm clear." That means that they are ready to go and able to give 100% participation today. Even that bit of information is valuable to know. It's also good to know that we are all working with friends who really care about us.

This few quiet minutes is also the forum where the team leader (like it or not, that's you, doctor) gets to set the emotional tone for the day. *A grumpy leader at the morning clearing will spend the day with a grumpy staff.* Also, a staff person, perhaps fresh from an argument at home, can have the whole course of their day changed by a few pleasant words here. The power that these few minutes exerts over the course of your day makes it difficult to overstate the importance of this time.

STEP 2. Structured communication exercise as part of our two-hour biweekly staff meetings. Our whole office meets every two weeks at 7:30 on Tuesday morning. The office is locked, with a sign stating that we are in conference and the door will be opened at exactly 9:30. Several chairs are set in the hallway. If patients come a little early they will be comfortable, as well as certain that we are aware of them and concerned with their well-being. (We even set an alarm clock for 9:25, so we never run over time and break our commitment to our patients.) The answering machine is left on, with a special message saying we will return all calls promptly at 9:30, so nothing will disturb us.

We rotate leadership of staff meetings among all staff, except doctors (we tend to talk too much anyway). A typed agenda has been handed out in advance to each team member, compiled from input all the staff has contributed over the two weeks since our last meeting. A blank agenda form has been posted on the lab wall since the end of our last meeting to make it convenient to jot down staff meeting ideas during the work day as they occur to people.

Each agenda item includes the name of the person who wishes to bring the topic up and how many minutes they need to discuss their concern. We time each item with a stopwatch, so we stay on schedule, and all topics get the time needed to properly consider them. Items not on the agenda are discussed at the end of the meeting, time permitting. Of course, staff are paid their normal salary to be here. We don't allow food (not even our beloved donuts) in the meeting. This is work!

Chapter 8 will be devoted to the staff meeting per se. Our concern here is with the communication part of the meeting, so if some of the portions of the meeting itself seem sketchy at this point, please don't be concerned. Chapter 8 will answer all your questions concerning details of our staff meeting process.

Now we come to our staff meetings' somewhat unique beginning. It's something we've done for years. I hate it! I hate getting ready for it. If it weren't so important to my growth as a person and our team development, I'd drop it like a hot rock! One more thing: this concept will scare you to death!

We call it our *communication exercise*. The exercise has two sections: incompletes and positives. Each staff member is *required* to have prepared at least two of each type of communication message to give. There is no maximum number of messages that can be given, but no one is allowed not to participate, because if nonparticipation were permitted, this whole concept wouldn't last two weeks. As essential to our office growth as this process is, I think you'll soon understand how difficult it is to perform. Sadly, it's tempting to abandon difficult things, even ones you know to be helpful. I believe any smoker or dieter can attest to this. That is why complete staff participation is mandated.

We begin with the *incompletes*. These are statements made by staff members describing something that has happened, that has left them with "feelings" that aren't complete. The *exact* situation that happened (with time, dates, and names) is stated, and how that event made the person now giving the message feel is expressed. All communications given must be carefully prepared in writing before the staff meeting begins. These messages are too sensitive and important for staff to just "wing it."

Once a communication is given, no dialog is allowed. Such discussions always end up with people trying to prove that they are "right" (which implies that someone else is "wrong"). These exercises have nothing to do with right or wrong. They are about a specific event that occurred, and how that incident made a staff member feel. Here's an example of an incomplete:

> Betsy: "John, when you left Thursday night before re-viewing the last patient's medical history and X-rays, I felt unsupported and concerned about your commitment."

You bet the doctor gets them! The whole idea is open, honest communication. If you allow yourself to get defensive and explain that you were in a hurry to give blood (and you may have had a noble excuse, but Betsy didn't know that and this is how she felt), then any chance for open and honest communication in your office has ended.

Are you scared yet? How many feelings do you think your staff has stored up that they'd like to share with you? Guess who gets the most incompletes? The doctor, at least at first. This trend to doctor-incompletes changes, as either the behavior of the doctor changes based on his new values and the feedback this system provides, or the entire plan is abandoned as repeated hypocritical behavior leads to more and more painful communication. Don't begin this system until you are sure your commitment to change and growth is sincere.

So, other than being crazy and masochistic, why would anyone choose to engage in such a process of flagellation? You choose to engage in these exercises so you can learn about yourself. You need to see how you are honestly perceived by your staff (and perhaps, your patients?), to show your commitment to growth as an individual and as a team member, to be honestly able to see your actions through another's eye, to decide, if *you choose*, to change, and to become close enough to your staff that you can tell each other the truth!

We all have feelings, and we can't control what feelings we have. However, we can make one vital decision: do we prefer to be honest or dishonest with these feelings? Dishonesty (as in being nice and just not mentioning what upset you, at least not to that person's face) is often easier, or seems so, until a staff member quits or goes into a rage. Once again our actions bear witness to the fact that easy is seldom best, and that honesty and courage are the best policies if we wish to thrive.

As I stated earlier, no dialog is allowed during our communication exercise, with one exception. The staff member giving the communication exercise can make a *request* for a change in the behavior of the staff member the communication is directed to. Let's go back to Betsy's incomplete and see how this might work. The request is stated immediately following the incomplete.

> Betsy: "John, I have a request. I request that you stay at the end of the day until all X-rays are read and medical histories have been reviewed."

People receiving requests have three options:

1. They can simply say, "Yes." They accept the request and commit in the future to adopt the suggested behavior.

2. They can say, "No." We much prefer a candid *no* to making a commitment that will not be kept. Such a broken commitment just adds to the team's frustration and reduces the staff member's credibility.

3. They can make a counteroffer or propose a second alternative. An example might be:

   John: "It's not always possible for me to stay late. I will make a commitment to remain in the office when I can, and on evenings when I'm unable to stay, to inform you before we see the last patient, so you will be aware that I have to leave."

The person who made the original request (Betsy), can now say, "Yes," "No," or counteroffer again. Almost always a solution is achieved, because we share a common purpose and are merely seeking the best possible way to arrive at this common goal. Even in the cases where no agreement can be reached, both parties now understand the other person's situation and point of view. Not infrequently we find the injured feelings were the result of an honest misunderstanding which the communication exercise allows us to clear up.

Again, no dialog outside the three choices outlined above is allowed. The rest of the staff is not allowed to speak. At the end of a staff meeting, concern about a decision reached can be raised, but the rules during the communication exercise itself are strict. If you are lax on these rules prohibiting discussion (and human nature being what it is, people will want to jump in and discuss the topics that are raised), you'll see the system break down to squabbling and self-defense. Neither is compatible with growth.

I believe you can see how consistent with our philosophy such honest communication is. We accept the short-term discomfort both by sharing our honest feelings and listening as others share theirs. The long-term gain is the creation of a relationship based on openness and honesty that is possible because all the people in our group work in an atmosphere of high trust.

The initiation of this exercise requires great courage from the doctor. You not only have to participate in the exercise, you have to set the example, if you wish to work with friends. You must accept the comments given to you in a positive manner as the potential tools for your personal growth that they are. *Any show of defensiveness on your part will end the honest communication given to you by the staff.* To achieve a committed team that pulls together unselfishly, honesty is the way. Did you think a thing of such value would be easy?

The *positives* are both easier to accept and explain. Each staff member recalls at least two things that have occurred which left them with positive feelings toward another staff person. In our office, this is often somebody being thanked for bringing food, but whatever the event was, it's nice to take the time to say thanks.

An example here would be:

> John: "Betsy, when you stayed over your lunch time to reseat a temporary crown I felt teamed and supported. You showed what a true commitment to our purpose looks like. Thanks!"

I tend to be a critical person. That is my nature, but it's not what I wish to be. For me, the effort to concentrate on the positive in my fellow workers is as critical as anything I do in the office or out. I never have less than four positives to contribute personally (two are required), and I'm much more likely to have eight.

There is a school of management that talks about how important it is to catch your people doing something right, and celebrate. We often practice dentistry in a negative environment. A patient with 31 healthy teeth often hears only of the one other, the tooth that has a problem. Here is our chance to celebrate the positive things in life. If you want behavior repeated, *reward it!* You especially, doctor, as the visionary and leader, must make a determined effort to "accentuate the positive."

The last step of our communication exercise is the opportunity for each of us to hug each member of the staff. It isn't required. Some staff choose to shake hands or ignore the whole thing and go to the bathroom. These choices are accepted by the staff, but it has been my experience that such a choice is often a signal that something is wrong. In the past a staff member who chose not to hug or shake hands consistently usually meant that I would soon be dusting off my help-wanted ads.

The power of these communication sessions, beyond their ability to forge a team of shared value and to encourage individual growth is that they will lead to changes in individual staff member's behavior.

If I personally take a staff person aside and discuss with them behavior I feel not in the best interest of our team—well, that is my opinion. If that same staff member is given seven incompletes from seven different team members about the same situation, it is very hard for anyone to ignore such feedback. One of two things will soon occur:

1. The behavior in question will change

2. The staff member will realize that due to an honest difference in values, our office is not the place for him or her to be at this time

STEP 3. Individual consultations between each staff member and the doctor. We have these meetings on a quarterly schedule. They probably should be held more often, but of all the communication steps, these are the most time consuming for the doctor both in preparation and in holding the individual meetings themselves.

Before we set down together, both the staff member and doctor fill out identical forms, in writing. When we do meet, in a quiet and private setting, we have at least 30 minutes of uninterrupted time available. The first thing we do is exchange these already-filled-out forms, and take a moment to read each other comments.

The first part of the form asks both the doctor and staff person to separately list the things we feel the staff person is doing extraordinarily well. We share our perceptions of these positive observations. This is a pleasant way for both of us to begin our meeting, and often positive contributions are mentioned that the other party hadn't been fully aware of.

The next section of the form instructs us to list specific goals that we both feel should be worked on by that staff person. After comparing each other's lists, agreement is reached on one or two goals we feel need immediate attention. We write these mutually agreed-upon goals down on both our copies of the form, and each sign them. These "contracts" are placed in the employee's permanent personnel file.

At the next individual consultation, an identical form is filled out before we begin, but previous to exchanging these new forms, we evaluate how the staff person has done on the mutually agreed-upon goals from our last meeting. We normally adjust staff salaries every six months. Staff people who haven't kept their commitments, as agreed to in writing at these consultations, are not eligible for raises. Of course, the more commitments made and kept, the greater the increase in remuneration.

Often I get the most value from these individual discussions after the formal meeting part has ended. Despite our years of communication exercises, there remain some topics so delicate that they can only be shared on a one-to-one basis. Often I'll hear the same concern from several people. This allows me to deal with a problem (usually involving one individual) before I would have even known it existed without this opportunity.

A FORMULA FOR DRAMATIC IMPROVEMENT

Having done these practice building exercises for years, I realize full well their cost in time, money, effort, and discomfort. (One reason we exchange written ideas in our individual consultations is because I used to fail to address the things I most wanted and needed to discuss when face to face. My discomfort level at times overcame my commitment.)

I hope that the advantages inherent in these systems are readily apparent to you now. I would like to caution you to be very patient, yet firm, in working to get your staff involved in this process. Patience is only fair as they have not gone through the value clarification process that you are experiencing. They must first learn what your vision is, then see if it is consistent with their personal values.

At first staff will probably believe that if they ignore all this, the whole thing will go away. How many other "brilliant ideas" have you brought to the office over the years that were eventually abandoned? If you haven't made the critical effort of clarifying your own values before this communication exercise was begun, this will be another concept to disappear.

All you need to convince them of your sincerity is a consistent effort on your part. With time, that will banish any doubts.

You must accept and be willing to face the fact that you will probably have staff turnover as a result of these policies. The length of time people have been with you has little to do with their acceptance of your vision. You may find the staff person who has been with you "forever," that you can't live without, may be the one to leave. Whoever leaves, they will take a lot of their personal as well as office turmoil with them. Turmoil is the broth created when people with varied values attempt to work together.

We've discussed why these staff changes occur and that it is nothing to feel sad about. This is just a part of the process of people seeking to find an environment consistent with their personal values. Be aware of the fact that even the staff that stays and is committed to the team vision you have developed will struggle. I'd strongly recommend sharing all or part of this book with them to help them in the transition.

Would you give anything to have a supportive, creative team? If you're tired of the way things are in your office and life, here's a formula for dramatic improvement. Like most worthwhile change, this will hurt. Change always does. To me the price is insignificant compared to the value received.

You'll make a lot more money in this "new" office. You'll have a lot more patients drawn by the positive feelings that are so evident there. (It's sad that a positive atmosphere is so rare that it attracts such attention.) The habits of open, honest, and caring communication will carry over to your relationships with family and friends. But I predict the most significant change will be a renewed interest and joy in your profession: a profession of people working together to help others, with a team committed to mutual growth, to the best possible care for your clients, and to having *fun!*

CHAPTER 8

---◆---

STAFF MEETINGS

I fully realize that staff meetings have existed since people had to use foot pedals to supply power to the handpiece. (I'm not that old, I just read about it.) I'd guess there are as many different ways to conduct staff meetings as there are dental offices. The differences in the forms of the meetings should occur because both the *objectives* of the staffings and the *collective values* of each team that meets are unique.

I want to describe our staff meetings in detail, so you can see exactly how the *particular structure we have adopted is consistent with our values and goals within our office*. As you read this description, please review in your mind how the structure, format, and policies we employ in our staff meetings coincide with our philosophy. What you should observe is that the form (of our meetings) follows the desired function.

Staff meetings are the instruments that turn "your" office into "our" office. It is also in these meetings that we unleash the *creative potential of the staff as a whole*. We perform these tasks of legerdemain by encouraging the entire staff to become involved in the creative and problem-solving tasks of running the office. It is during this act of creation that ownership of the office evolves.

Using techniques like brainstorming and piggybacking (which I'll describe fully later in this chapter), we also illustrate that the potential achievements of a group of people working together creatively is exponential to what the same individuals working separately could hope to perform.

So as we proceed with the description of our meetings, please bear in mind:

1. Our staff meetings, in their every form and facet, should consistently mirror our office philosophy.

2. As we labor as a team, ownership of the office (as opposed to simply being a place of employment) is created and nurtured in all the staff. This is a byproduct of the creative process. Wouldn't it be great to work with a team whose every member feels as committed personally to the things you are trying to accomplish in the office as you are?

3. Note the creative potential that is unleashed when people united by a common set of values work together to solve mutual problems. Attempt also to be aware of the tenor or mood of the meetings, one of trust and enthusiasm. Your office will now do things routinely that you never thought possible, due to the forces inherent in such synergism.

We have discussed the communication exercise done in our staff meetings in the previous chapter. No further discussion of that vital step of our team development will be included here. A few of the staff-meeting items mentioned briefly in Chapter 7 will be discussed again here to enable us to now fully flesh out these topics. Also, I'd like this chapter to contain all the information on staff meetings so it can serve as an easy-access reference source for your office team to work with.

Let's begin by looking at a copy of an actual agenda from a past staff meeting in our office. There was nothing noteworthy about this particular meeting. I would like to present it to you as an example of our typical staff meeting agenda and use it as the basis for our discussion.

STAFF MEETING AGENDA

Date: _____
Leader: Kathy
Secretary: Betsy

1. PURPOSE

2. Agreements: a) not to subgroup b) is everyone safe?

3. Communication Exercises
   A. Incompletes
   B. Positives
   C. Hugs

4. Requests
   Betsy—assist. scheduled later with John—3 minutes
   Carol—Vacuum—2 minutes
   Carol and Kathy—changes on treatment complete—notes in progress —
      insurance—2 minutes
   Vickey—X-ray on hygiene schedule—2 minutes
   Carol—charges performed off under wrong doctor—5 minutes
   Carol—emergency patients—scheduled for NP—Pano/fmx not
      estimated—2 minutes
   John—senior programs in line—2 minutes
   John—policy on charity—stress true expense of the gift—3 minutes
   John—uniforms all set—1 minute
   John—pink card, are we filling one out for everyone who makes financial
      arrangements—even for a week?—2 minutes
   John—comments on Mitch and Lisa—2 minutes
TARGETS:
   Are all medical histories getting new stickers on them?
   Lowell, are your supper breaks OK?
   Are we scheduling Lowell's long op on Monday and Wednesday?
   Are we watching Lowell's schedule on Thur. that we are only scheduling
      hyg checks after 5:00 P.M.?
   Front office: are we getting pink cards/truth lending?

5. Agree NOT to Subgroup
Date of next meeting:
Leader: VICKEY
Secretary: KATHY

Here you have an exact reproduction of one of our previous staff meeting agendas, complete with typos, inexact punctuation, misspelling and abbrev. I wanted to reproduce it in this fashion to show it as a working document. Many of the notes contained in this document were jotted down during the course of a busy day and are in a shorthand that is intelligible only to the writers (and sometimes not even to them). We don't take off points for form, but rather award them on the basis of commitment and creative thought.

The leader of this particular meeting, Kathy, has taken this agenda down from the lab wall, where a blank form was hung immediately after the last staff meeting by that meeting's leader. She has typed this amazingly rough document into the rough (but at least now readable) document you have just reviewed. This agenda is passed out to all staff members on Monday, the day before our meeting.

The leadership of the meeting is rotated among all our staff, except doctors (who tend to prolixity, remember?). We based our sequence of leaders on the age of the staff (showing great creativity and ingenuity). You may go by seniority—I'd definitely avoid weight as a system to establish the order of your leaders—but in some fashion, get a sequential list of people and rotate the leadership of the meetings through that list.

The secretary of today's staffing takes notes during the meeting, types them, and then passes them out the day of our meeting to all the staff. The secretary is simply the leader from our last meeting (we'd never survive two lists). The notes are a helpful reminder to all of us as to exactly what conclusions we reached on each of the topics discussed. They also identify in writing who made what commitments and by what date that promised labor is to be completed. The notes are also useful to help us review and prepare for the next meeting in two weeks.

Our purpose has been discussed at length. It is read out loud before the beginning of each staff meeting by that meeting's leader. I believe that it sets the proper tone for the endeavor we are about to undertake by reminding us of the shared beliefs that have brought us together. We all know the purpose, so why read it? As we discussed earlier, a leader gets a vision, and then *repeats it!* Our purpose is the physical and verbal manifestation of our collective vision.

The agreements listed on the agenda are an integral part of our office and the beliefs we share. For our first agreement, we all commit vocally and in turn not to subgroup. Subgrouping is talking about other team members in a negative manner when they are not present. We state out loud that we will refrain from doing this at the beginning and at the end of each staff meeting. We state this twice, one person at a time and out loud, because it is so difficult to avoid talking behind another's back, and also because it is vitally important to our team's success that we do refrain from this most destructive behavior.

There is a second commitment inherent in our agreement not to subgroup. If someone breaks the agreement and subgroups to me, I agree to take them to the person they need to talk to (i.e., the person they were talking about) and initiate a face-to-face conversation between them. Then something constructive may result from whatever the difficulty was that lead to the subgrouping originally.

Say that Kathleen, our hygienist, comes to me in the lab complaining that she can never find her assistant, Vickey, when she needs her. (We use the real names of our staff members here, since none of us are so innocent as to need protecting.) Time is wasted during the search process, patients have to wait, and (probably worst of all), we have an unhappy hygienist. (Remember your Shakespeare, "Hell hath no fury like a waiting hygienist," or some such thing.) This outrage occurs despite a solemn promise from Vickey to stay within earshot of Kathleen's strident tones.

In my youth I would have met with both these ladies and rather pedantically lectured and scolded. I would have provided them with a solution to *their* problem. They would have resented my interference, and the solution wouldn't have worked anyway, because I am neither a hygienist or an assistant. What do I know about their problems? Except it would have become *my* problem. I would have made it so by my act of attempting to solve it for them. I would have taken that monkey off their backs and placed him four square on mine. The last I need or want is more problems! (Does any of this scenario sound familiar, doctor?)

Today, the new enlightened John (at least "lightened" in the sense of fewer monkeys on my back) would take Kathleen by the hand (though considering her emotional state by this time, "claw" might be more correct) and take her wherever Vickey is hiding. I'd say, "You two need to talk. Use my office and please do it now." The problem is now in the correct hands/claws to solve it, and the monkey is off my back. (The monkey is a figure of speech, not to be confused with any of my staff.)

(The jocular tone of this description is typical of our office, a place where friends work together. We tease and kid a lot. I am called John, not doctor, by my staff, and on my bad days, sometimes a lot worse. We joke and have fun with each other. The inexplicable increase in skin showing through where hair once reigned, as well as my latent pregnancy, now seemingly at the four-month point, are fair and frequent cause for comment. People working together for a common purpose are able to kid each other. I mention this only as I felt some monkeys may have been offended by reference to them looking like my staff. If they were, I can only say, "Lighten up!")

If a problem identified by subgrouping is critical to the office, I may choose to check later and see if or how it was resolved. It may need to be brought up in a staff meeting for our full group's discussion. Most subgrouping is of a personal, rather than procedural, nature and needs to be solved in private by the parties involved.

I can think of no activity more destructive to the team well-being than subgrouping. It destroys both team morale and interpersonal relationships. Patients are aware of the low-trust atmosphere engendered by such behavior. Somehow the unkind words spoken behind someone's back unfailingly find their way to the individual being besmirched. No positive gain results, but a lot of negative garbage comes from such behavior.

That said, and with our two agreements not to indulge in this pastime, is our office free of such behavior? *No!* We are human (most of us at least). This seems a behavior that, despite all our efforts, humans are prone to do. We do often find ourselves stopping in mid-subgroup, as our commitment is recalled. I hope our agreement significantly reduces this behavior among us.

If we can't stop subgrouping completely, are we hypocritical to keep making this commitment? I don't know about you, but if I gave up everything I wasn't perfect at, I'd have a lot of time on my hands! Remember, it's the honest effort, not the results that are most important.

Our second "agreement" consists of asking the question, "Is everyone safe?" We don't get much response to this query today, but in the early days of our staff meeting, it was frequently answered in the negative.

Safe means that you are able to participate in the staff meeting at a 100% level. Said another way, nothing is blocking you from this goal. If there is a problem that makes you nervous (not safe), let's get it out in the open and deal with it before our meeting begins. We can't be a true team unless all of us are involved in the meeting completely.

I'm always delighted when someone isn't safe. It means some staff member is courageously about to open a difficult, emotional topic. You can trust that this will be a key issue related closely to the growth and overall well-being of the office. If we had no purpose, it would be impossible to reassure a person that we support them in this as-yet-unnamed poser. As it is, we can promise them if their subject is consistent with our office purpose, they will indeed have our collective support. Usually this reassurance, that if their cause is intended to improve the office we will all support them, is the difference between a vital issue being dealt with, and the easier alternative of just not mentioning it. As always, the tougher path leads to growth.

To summarize, someone isn't safe when they feel unable to deal with an important issue during the course of our meeting. We do whatever is needed by people to make them safe and allow them to proceed. You could call this emotional hand-holding, but the usual reason that someone is unsafe is that they have had the courage to bring up an important issue none of the rest of us is brave enough to raise.

These agreements are followed by the communication exercise we've covered in the proceeding chapter. Note as we go along how consistently the values illuminated by the communication exercise fit in with the purpose behind all the other things we're doing in the staff meeting. Can you see our underlying philosophy behind each of the steps involved?

The reading of our office purpose, our agreements, and the completion of our communication exercise is the basic team-building portion of our staff meeting. The *requests* are the nuts-and-bolts of each meeting. This is where the process of working together to solve problems to our mutual benefit occurs. This is also where the creative power of many minds working as one is realized.

Don't make an effort to study the actual requests on our agenda. They will mean nothing to you. Do note how many different members of our staff have contributed requests. This is one small indication of the team concept, all of us raising issues that are important to the whole. Certainly, some people are more instrumental in raising questions than others during any given meeting. That doesn't mean other staff can't be influential in helping to solve them. Let's take one example and recreate the process that went into working through that particular problem.

One request states: "John—senior programs in line—2 minutes." This is a request for a quick check on the status of the programs we developed for Senior Smile Month. In a previous meeting the topic of what our office could do to improve the dental health of seniors was raised. Let's use this subject to illustrate the process of brainstorming.

First, we *commit* as a staff to develop a program for seniors. We all agree such a topic is consistent with our purpose and worthy of our efforts. Then the creative brainstorming process begins. One person acts as a secretary and records ideas on a large blackboard, visible to all. Brainstorming involves a quick throwing out of ideas having to do with our selected topic, in this case Senior Smile Month. During this first stage of brainstorming, no criticism or censorship of ideas is allowed. Every concept is simply recorded as stated by our secretary. Piggyback-ing is encouraged. This is "hopping on" an existing idea with an additional related idea. The more ideas thrown out, no matter how seemingly far-fetched, the greater our creative possibilities.

One of the ideas suggested involved giving a party for seniors. Piggy-back ideas would be to have a dance, to wear costumes, to have a drawing for dental health items, and so on. Eventually our creative ideas wane or we just decide we have a sufficient number of ideas to proceed with.

Now we begin the process of carefully analyzing each idea. Both criticism, as well as additional piggybacking to further develop the original concepts are encouraged. Some ideas, upon critical reflection, are now abandoned. Others seem to have promise. To develop these ideas, specific people are assigned to specific tasks to be completed by (you guessed it) a specific date. These people, assignments, and dates are recorded by this meeting's secretary in our staff meeting notes for later followup.

We use only volunteers to follow up on our varied projects. The people who pursue these ideas need to be committed to their success. This is the concept of ideas having *champions* to stand up for them, as discussed in the outstanding book *In Search of Excellence*. A champion is someone who really believes in an idea and will do all in his/her power to see it succeed. Such determination and dedication to a worthy project by any of your staff should merit praise and rewards. Remember, if you want behavior repeated, reward it.

At the next staff meeting, we will review the information gathered by these champions and begin to make decisions concerning our course of action. Again, as the problems associated with any given project may dictate, volunteers will be assigned to follow up on specific tasks by specific dates. These dates are selected by the people doing the work, but once recorded, we expect them to abide by their self-imposed time commitment.

What if a commitment isn't kept? In such a case, some judgment will be required. First, get all the facts. There may have been a reason it was impossible for the person who made the commitment to complete the task in a timely manner. But, if the job "just didn't get done," a problem exists. Perhaps the person originally assigned to the task will request another chance and set a new date. The team will have to decide if he/she is still the right person to champion this project. Perhaps additional assistance is needed.

In our office it's very unusual when an assignment isn't completed on time. All commitments, the people who made them, and the dates *they chose* to have it completed are all recorded in the staff meeting notes, a copy of which is given to every staff member. Failure to keep a promise is a rare, but very serious occurrence for us. If any people are allowed to not do their share, or if assignments are made and not followed up on, soon the entire system will have ceased to exist. Continuity and commitment are the lifeblood of our staff meetings.

I trust this illustration of how one request was dealt with in the venue of a typical staff meeting in our office will be adequate to begin your team on its own process of problem-solving. Once you have formed a team, and someone has identified a problem, I'm sure you'll quickly work out a problem-solving method that will be ideal for your unique needs.

Targets are the mechanisms we use to ensure our staff's continuity. A target is a goal that we had created in a previous meeting. We review targets to make sure we hit the goal. Targets are not projects in the development stage, but rather completed ones. We may need to reassess the status of a developed system or possibly even drop it from future consideration if we can see no value resulting from our efforts. The champion of each idea will report on its progress, but all of us must review the status of the job and judge its worthiness. Wasting valuable staff time on a project with no appreciable payback is avoided by each task being analyzed by the whole staff at each meeting. We want to avoid wasting assets from someone doggedly pursuing a project they believe in that less-involved people can see is not worth the effort it requires to bring to fruition.

Our next topic isn't on the formal agenda. If we have time, after the targets have been checked, we ask people if there are any other topics they wish to discuss. This could be an idea that was thought of too late for placing on the agenda or an inspiration that occurred during the course of the staffing. If no time is left, the topic can be noted on the new blank agenda form, placed on our lab wall immediately at the end of this meeting by the leader, for discussion at our next staffing.

We now all recommit again out loud and one at a time, not to subgroup.

The last thing we do before adjourning is for each of us to state out loud that we are *clear*. This means nothing is left over from our discussions that needs to be said. Someone may wish to briefly thank a fellow team member for their efforts during the meeting. A possible misunderstanding may need to be cleared up. Some upset feelings remaining from an earlier topic may need to be expressed. Several staff members may need to commit to a short meeting later that day to finalize a topic dealt with during the main meeting. The point of the clearing process is to be sure no loose ends remain at the conclusion of the meeting.

We go directly from these meetings to treat our patients. The atmosphere we leave the meeting with should be one of excitement and a sense of oneness created by our work completed together. Stating that we are clear and 100% ready to proceed with our tasks of the day ahead assures that this is the case. Again, I believe it is incumbent on the doctor as the team leader, that no matter what the tenor of the staff meeting, the team leaves with a positive feeling about themselves.

This is the end of our biweekly, full-team meeting. There remains to discuss separate staff meetings that take place between just the front-office people and just the hygiene staff. These are held once a month and immediately follow the regular staff meeting. They will usually last about 40 minutes. Holding these department meetings keeps us from having to tie up the entire staff's time with matters that don't directly affect them, but are only relevant to people in particular departments of our office. Issues that do concern the entire staff raised at these submeetings are simply placed on the agenda for the next regularly scheduled full-staff meeting, to be dealt with then by the entire team.

We have no communication process in either of these department meetings. All the people involved have just left our whole staff meeting, so there is no need to repeat the team-building and communication exercises we've all just completed. In the departmental meetings, we rotate leaders, just as in the previous meeting and also have a written and timed agenda. This is posted between meetings in a place convenient for the people involved in these particular departments.

Meeting with only your most direct co-workers, be it front office or hygiene, helps improve relationships for these teams within teams. Topics can be discussed that would be less than comfortable in front of the combined staff. Both hygiene and the front office have their own set of monitors they have developed and keep for their own personal information (and to keep me up to date on what is happening in their areas). Their special monitors are reviewed and discussed during these meetings.

In the past a few meetings were held with just chairsides and doctors. We decided that most of the issues that arise between us could be dealt with on the spot. We can also use our regular staff meeting to discuss chairside-doctor concerns more fully, if need be. My newest chairside has been with us three years. If your situation is different, with new personnel or procedures being adopted, you may choose to have a staffing with the chairsides and doctors on a regular basis. I would base the decision on having chairside staff meetings on your assessment of your office need for improved communication and teamwork among these vital members of your staff.

I know the time, effort, and expense for all these activities seem staggering, if not downright prohibitive. Let me remind you once again of our office production goals: *high net.* To achieve this requires a committed *team* effort. I doubt a single doctor, whatever the number of auxiliaries he/she may employ, could net $2,000 a day based on his own energy and creative ideas if the office doesn't truly function as a team. I certainly couldn't. Even if this were possible, it would be an exhausting, as well as lonely way to exist.

The rewards garnered from these staff-meeting efforts should be partly financial, but when you consider the effort involved and decide whether the reward justifies the expense, don't overlook the much more difficult-to-measure intangibles. The sense of teamwork, honesty, and friendship in our working environment has inestimable worth to me. I also deeply believe in the need for all of us to experience growth as individuals. Consider all these facets carefully as you decide on making a commitment of the magnitude needed to create this system and make it work.

The effort required on your part for true team development will be tremendous. Your commitment to such a system must be long term. Don't expect either you or your staff to instantly and unanimously grasp all of this information. What starts you on this course and keeps you motivated are clearly defined values and goals, first by the team leader and then by the developing team in the manner we've just discussed. Without these clear values, these ideas have no chance of success. With them, financial rewards and the joys of creating and interacting with a committed team await.

CHAPTER 9

FINDING THE RIGHT MEMBERS FOR YOUR TEAM

Nothing is more critical to the ultimate success of a dental office than the selection of the individuals that comprise the dental team. The creation of an inspiring vision and even the most vivid sharing of it will do no good if the people who form your team are, by their nature, not receptive to the particular values and goals this vision entails. It is possible to make some minor changes in the behavior of team members through training and sharing of the vision of your office. It is not possible to change the basic character of the individuals you employ. The key to finding the right people to fulfill your office vision is to:

1. Clearly identify the values in others that your professional vision requires for the development of the office of your dreams

2. Create a hiring process that when followed will make the virtues you esteem obvious in the people you are evaluating

3. Consistently follow that process in staff selection

No amount of effort or patience in staff training nor the most sophisticated of staff meetings can replace the essential task of hiring the right person in the first place.

Let's examine a hypothetical situation (which, of course, really happened to me) and see if we can illustrate these points more clearly. Suppose you have a chairside that has been employed in your office for a number of years. She is both punctual and reliable. She works hard at her job and is dexterous and efficient. Before you clarified your values and set goals for what you envisioned your practice to become, you were very pleased with her performance.

A significant part of the values you have identified deal with relating to the patient as a whole person, not just a mouth containing teeth to be worked on. To reach these objectives will require the development of a high-trust relationship that allows for a meaningful dialog between your staff and patients. This type of meaningful conversation will enable both you and your staff to help patients clarify their personal values in regards to their own dental health. Thus, through this personal relationship, your office is better able to help the patients you treat both select and achieve the level of dental health appropriate for them.

In this new awareness, you begin to notice that your prized assistant, the pinnacle of chairside efficiency, is rather cold and abrupt with patients. She seems annoyed by questions and likes to hurry clients out of the operatory to prepare the treatment area for the next procedure.

Your other chairside has never been outstandingly efficient. She seems to like to visit with the patients and just doesn't work as quickly as her fellow assistant. This pattern of behavior used to annoy you on busy days, but now you notice how the patients seem to frequently ask her questions. For some reason they ask her about their dental needs, even after you have left the treatment area, your scholarly explanation of needed care still hanging freshly in the vapors. In light of your newly identified values, you see that this knack of answering patient questions concerning proposed care is essential for the creation of the high-trust relationships you are trying to establish with your clients.

In this scenario we have identified a difference in values between the two staff people we've discussed. Depending on the criteria of excellence established by the team leader, *one* of these assistants will be judged as outstanding, and the other as wanting. But which individual is perceived to be outstanding is totally the opinion of the person doing the judging. What you must see is that neither person's actions are right or wrong, good or bad. They are simply behaving in a way consistent with their own personal values.

The first assistant we described values hard work and efficiency. She's not too comfortable with people, but prefers to concentrate her efforts on the performance of tasks. Her strengths are her ability to produce prodigious amounts of work and her reliability.

Our second staff person is a people person. She has good skills chairside, but she comes to work to be with people and help them, not simply to pass instruments. It is the conversation and company she enjoys. The work of assisting is something she tolerates while receiving her enjoyment from the people she is around.

I don't believe it is possible to transmute the characters of one assistant into the other, no matter how hard you try. I believe that an effort to change the nature of people leads only to frustration on the part of everyone involved. You have three choices in this situation.

1. You can continue as you have been and face the growing tensions that comes from conflicts in values and poor communication.

2. You can reassign the assistant whose values don't coincide with yours to a job that will accent her strengths and hide what you now perceive to be her weakness. Possibly a front office or clerical position requiring great concentration and accuracy with less patient interaction would make our hard-working, but not people-oriented team member once again a valued team member. For your "people person," maybe the ideal position would be in case presentation or the delicate job of collections that requires tact more than efficiency. One of these positions could be more suited to her natural temperament.

3. The third choice is to tell your staff member she is not the right person for the job she is in (she'll know already) and support her as she searches for another position where she very well may become that office's "star."

As you clarify your values, you may lose a "former star" in your office. This change is a normal part of growth. I only hope the two of you don't torture each other too long in a battle over whose values are best. Remember, values aren't correct or faulty, they just are. You own the office, so if employees don't share your values, it is they who must move on. These people are just as entitled to their beliefs as you are yours. Never allow yourself a feeling of superiority in the area of values. As you go through life and hopefully experience growth, your own values will continue to change. It makes no sense to attempt to rate something as ephemeral personal beliefs.

Now, as staff positions open up due to attrition, growth of the office, or your realization that you have staff members in your office that simply don't belong there, you are faced with the most critical of tasks. You must locate and hire people who already share your common values and thus will be able to commit to the vision your office has identified. How many present staff members you have to replace will simply reflect how distorted your office operations were before your own beliefs were clarified.

The system we use in our office for hiring staff is deliberate and demanding. It requires a lot of time and effort. In our office we have one staff member who has been with us since a few months after the office opened, 20 years ago. The average length of employment of our current staff is about six years. This average is decreased by the fact that the office has grown and so added additional staff members. My point is that the process of hiring the right people repays you many times over, because you won't have to begin the search for a new person again every three months, when you realize the last person you selected isn't going to work out. Also, there exists little conflict and a great deal of joy in working every day with people who share your beliefs and values.

Let us go carefully through all the steps that our hiring procedure entails. I assure you that every time we add staff, this is the exact process we follow, point by painstaking point. Let the complexity and detail of this process convince you of how important the selection of the right staff is to the success of our office.

Before we enter the hiring arena, allow me to beg your indulgence on one point. In all the years I have been in practice, I have had one male applicant for a position (he wasn't qualified). In this lengthy chapter I will refer to all applicants as females. I do this only to simplify the writing process. In my two years in the military, I am proud to say I served with many excellent male auxiliaries. I hope to see an increase in male ancillary staffing. We need all the good people we can get in our profession. Unfortunately where I practice I know of no males employed in any area offices.

The first and most critical step in our hiring process is to attract a large pool of outstanding applicants. We need our search process to reach out to people who share our values, no matter what field of employment they have previously worked in. We would like our efforts to yield applications from people who previously believed they would never consider working for a dentist. In our rural area, I seldom have more than two or three people apply with previous dental office experience or training. To allow us the greatest possible chance of finding the ideal person to join our team, we *must* recruit applicants from outside the normal group of individuals who might consider a dental office as a possible place of employment. For example, in the past, two people with teaching degrees have graced our office with their presence.

Our process of attracting new staff members revolves principally around help-wanted ads placed in every local paper within a 20-mile radius of our office. We have no dental assistants' association or assistant school near us to approach as a possible source of job applicants. If we were fortunate enough to have either resource available to us, they would be the first entities I would contact in my search for additional team members.

Anything you can do to increase the supply of potential staff members who apply for work with your team is good. There may well be opportunities for you to explore in your location that don't exist in ours.

Our staff has a standing offer of a $100 bonus if they identify a potential staff person to us that we hire. In the spirit of full disclosure, I must confess that this has not yet occurred. I personally keep my eyes open for patients, waitresses, bank tellers, or anyone else I feel may possess the qualities we esteem. I have never yet found an employee by this method either, but we continue to search in both these ways.

In our rural area the fact is that more than 90% of the applicant pool our office attracts comes from the help-wanted ad that follows. That means the makeup and character of the ad your office places is critical. This ad must accurately identify the *values* you seek in your future staff member. You wish for it to appeal to people who share similar beliefs to those you and your team hold. For our office, the following advertisement does this job. Your office ad will vary to reflect your own unique values.

DENTAL TEAM: Are you kind, compassionate, people-oriented, and motivated to succeed? We are seeking an exceptional person for our progressive office. We value superior organizational and administrative skills, and we focus on warmth, caring, and expert communication with our clients. We emphasize personal development through continuing education, full participation with the other members of our team, and high involvement with our clients. Although previous experience in dentistry is not essential, we believe that applicants should be career minded, personally stable, and health centered in their lifestyle. If you are searching for a real opportunity to grow and fulfill your potential, please send a complete résumé to Dr. John A. Wilde, D.D.S., P.C. 1610 Morgan Street, Keokuk, Iowa 52632.

Please place this in your paper for one week.
Thank you.
John A. Wilde D.D.S., P.C.

I'd like to point out two salient features of our ad. The first is that the entire description of the person we are searching for is based on values. The second is that we have none of the *normal* stuff usually listed about jobs in this ad. Nothing that says good hours, salary, or benefits. Our position provides all those things, but to state these facts about our available job won't appeal to the values held by the people we are trying to identify. We are not seeking to hire people whose main motivation to work is to obtain the "things" they are given for their job performance.

We seek people who are kind and compassionate to others. We want applicants who are already exceptional and want to grow. It's OK if they have worked in a dental office previously, but we're more concerned about their innate character. Do they share the values that we believe in and try to share with our clients? Would I hire a smoker? No. That behavior illustrates to me values not consistent with what our staff believes in.

We make compromises, of course. This ad is our best effort to identify the values that we all admire. We don't all live up to these values every moment of our lives, but they represent our goals. Do you see why value clarification is so essential before you can begin the hiring process? *For us, values are the hiring process.* In other words, in our office hiring consists of identifying the values we want in a new staff member and finding someone who shares those values. Once we find the right person, we'll be able to teach them to perform the job. This ad also keeps some folks away. The people whose only question about an available position is, How much does it pay? aren't attracted by this ad. We rarely have a smoker even apply. The two things we wish ideally to achieve through this publication are to:

1. Maximize the flow of applications from like-valued people

2. Minimize the applications from folks, no matter how delightful, who don't belong as employees in our office

Don't copy this ad. Set down with your team and create a statement that helps you to proceed in your own value-clarification process. Use the ad creation in a manner similar to the building of your purpose (which should be completed before the ad is created). Ask, "What do we want in this new staff member?" Not just what tasks must she perform, but what kind of a person do we seek? The answer to this question defines your ad.

Now that our ad has been placed, the résumés come rolling in. Depending on the local economy and time of year, we will receive between 30 and 70 applications. I review these applications personally. Some I eliminate out of hand. I get rid of the ones written in pencil or from recent high school graduates unless they identify something about themselves that really catches my eye. I enjoy the company of young people, but it is extremely rare to find a 20-year-old who has a clearly thought-out set of values. I am lenient in this stage of the process however. Anyone I eliminate now will be dropped from further consideration. If there is *any chance*, in my estimation, of the candidate having potential, I pass them on to the next step in our hiring procedure.

This next step in our hiring process is performed by a staff member. It consists of a patterned telephone interview. This is always done by a senior staff member, usually the most senior in the department to which we will be adding the new employee. I say "patterned interview" because the same employee asks the same questions to each applicant. This is a time-consuming task, and we have to free the staff person doing the telephone interviews from the tasks that would normally occupy her day for a considerable amount of time. We must allow her whatever time is required to carefully accomplish this important part of our hiring process. Take a moment and review the form used for this step of our selection process.

TELEPHONE INTERVIEW

Name: _____

Address: _____

Phone: Home _____ Office _____

How long have you lived at your current address? _____

How often have you moved in the last 5 years? _____

Do you have reliable transportation available?_____ What? _____

What hours are you available to work? ☐ Full-time ☐ Part-time
☐ Evenings ☐ Saturday

What salary do you expect? _____

When would you be available to start working? _____

Are you currently employed? _____ Where? _____

Can we contact them?_____ What is your job title? _____

How long have you worked there? _____

Previous job held _____ Reason for leaving _____

If employed, how long? _____

Have you been absent many days during the past years? _____
    Why? _____

Do you smoke? _____

Is there a reason why you couldn't pass a physical exam? _____

Is there someone you consider your dentist? _____

What condition do you consider your teeth and gums to be in? _____
_____

How often do you visit a dentist? _____

What was the highest grade you completed in school? _____

Have you had any college or advanced training? _____

What hobbies or interests do you have? _____
_____

Are you a member of any civic, professional, or social organization?_____
_____

What are your plans for the next 5 years? _____

TELEPHONE IMPRESSIONS: ☐ Excellent ☐ Good ☐ Fair ☐ Poor
    Capacity to communicate: _____
    Voice: _____
    Clarity of expression: _____
    Ease of expression: _____

The staff person conducting the interview needs to take a few minutes to explain to the applicant the purpose of this call. The tone she sets with the applicant should be friendly and relaxed, even fun. The questions start with requests for some simple facts that we probably already have available from the résumé the applicant has sent us. We need to allow a little time for the candidates to relax and be at their best. Answering these early factual questions provides this opportunity.

I think the reason for us wanting to acquire most of the factual information is self-evident. You will see as we proceed that we concentrate a lot of our attention on the dental awareness of the applicant. In my past experience, hiring someone with no history of valuing good oral health has proven to be a big mistake. No matter how strong any applicant's other features may be, if she has been to the dentist only once in the last five years and that for treatment of a toothache, she has almost no chance of being invited for a personal interview.

Some of you may feel that this deficiency in dental value by the applicant can be overcome by proper education if the candidate has other excellent qualities. This may be true, but it has decidedly *not* been the case in my experience. I believe the questions concerning the applicant's dental history are really inquiries into this individual's personal values and feelings concerning her level of commitment to personal well-being.

Hobbies are important if you wish to hire a chairside. Most people with good eye-hand coordination find ways to use this skill. It may be knitting, sewing, or playing the piano, but there is usually some indication of this innate coordination in the applicant's choice of hobbies. (Personally, I like to read. If you saw an amalgam I had carved, I think you would agree this supports my point that eye-hand coordination will be revealed by a choice of activities selected. At least I do turn my own pages.)

I like to employ people who are involved socially. They are the "people-oriented" kind of staff we are searching for. Leadership in organizations is even more impressive, since it shows they are committed to these activities, and are acknowledged as leaders by their peers.

As for their future plans, if they wish to have a baby or return to school, this job isn't for them. The best assistant in the world does me no good if she is no longer employed in my office.

All this information is helpful, but we gather a lot of the same data on the application form we'll discuss next. The *critical* function of this interview is the *personal impression made by the applicant on the staff person conducting the interview.* If the applicants come off badly in the staff's appraisal, they have little chance of proceeding in the hiring process. If they sound flat, dull, and lifeless on the phone now, I certainly don't want them to represent our office.

The most essential section of the telephone interview that I depend on to help me in the selection process is the *telephone impression section* at the very end of the form. It is here that I ask my staff for that critical intangible: their judgment. The impression made by the applicant on my skilled staff member during this lengthy conversation is much more important to me than any data we may have recorded.

Candidates who pass this stage of the hiring process are invited to our office and asked to fill out our personal record form. The applicant completes it in our reception room during office hours. If at all possible, the filling out of this form is scheduled at a time when the same staff person who did the phone interview is present. Thus the applicant is greeted by an "old friend."

When the applicants present themselves to complete the personal record form, they are again evaluated by the staff. I believe this evaluation to be more meaningful if done by the same individual who has engaged in the phone conversation with them recently. When they arrived to fill out the application, were they pleasant and friendly? Did they have nice smiles? Were their appearances neat and professional? We don't look to hire beauty queens, but we do want staff members who represent our values of good health and show a positive self-image by looking neat and professional. How attractive God happened to make them doesn't matter to us at all. We are concerned with the *values* they display in their behavior and demeanor. (I have a dentist friend in his fifties who, every time I visited his office, had another 20-year-old curvaceous blond assistant. I once asked him if he does a job interview or just asks them to send him a snapshot of their hips. I yield to no man in my admiration of curvaceous hips, but this plays no part in our staff selection process.)

I can't overstress the value I place on staff evaluation of candidates. The formal interview process that I conduct is stressful and takes place in an artificial environment. So often the true qualities of a person, good or bad, are more accurately revealed in the less-formal relations with my staff. Applicants will let their hair down and ask questions of the staff they would never dream of asking in the interview. This knowledge gained through the perception of experienced team members is priceless in the selection process.

PERSONAL RECORD FORM

Please be as complete as possible. All information you give here will be held in *strict confidence.*

Name_____ Date_____

Address _____

Previous address _____

Home phone_____ Social Security Number _____

Earnings expected _____

Work experience: Please start with your present or most recent position.

I. Employer _____

   Address _____

   Business phone _____ Employed from_____ to _____

   Kind of work_____ Your title _____

   Nature of your work _____

   Skills acquired _____

   Salary or salary range _____

   Supervisory responsibility_____ Immed. superior _____

   What do you enjoy best about your job? _____

   _____

   What do you enjoy least about your job? _____

   _____

   Reason for leaving (or desiring a change)? _____

   _____

II. Employer _____

   Address _____

   Business phone _____ Employed from_____ to _____

   Kind of work_____ Your title _____

   Nature of your work _____

   Skills acquired _____

   Salary or salary range _____

   Supervisory responsibility_____ Immed. superior _____

   What do you enjoy best about your job? _____

   _____

What do you enjoy least about your job? _____

_____

Reason for leaving (or desiring a change)? _____

_____

III. Employer _____

Address _____

Business phone _____ Employed from_____ to _____

Kind of work_____ Your title _____

Nature of your work _____

Skills acquired _____

Salary or salary range _____

Supervisory responsibility_____ Immed. superior _____

What do you enjoy best about your job? _____

_____

What do you enjoy least about your job? _____

_____

Reason for leaving (or desiring a change)? _____

_____

Other positions held:

a. company b. city	a. type of work b. name of superior	Date a. began b. left	Earnings a. start b. left	Reasons for leaving
a. _____	_____	_____	_____	_____
b. _____	_____	_____	_____	_____
a. _____	_____	_____	_____	_____
b. _____	_____	_____	_____	_____
a. _____	_____	_____	_____	_____
b. _____	_____	_____	_____	_____

Indicate by number any of the above employers you do not wish contacted. ___

_____

ACTIVITIES AND INTERESTS

Membership in civic, professional, or social organizations _____

_____

What hobbies interest you? _____

Why did you apply for this position? _____

_____

In what way do you feel qualified for this position? _____

What are your plans for the future? _____
_____

Why do you work? _____
What starting salary would you expect? _____
What income would you desire to enable you to live as you would like to live?
_____

Please list three references:

Names	Addresses	Phone numbers
1. _____	_____	_____
_____	_____	_____
2. _____	_____	_____
_____	_____	_____
3. _____	_____	_____
_____	_____	_____

PHYSICAL DATA

List any serious illness, operation, accident, or nervous disorder you have had
with approximate dates _____
What allergies do you have? _____
What medications do you take? _____
What brand of cigarettes do you smoke?_____ Why? _____
Would a job that required you to be on your feet all day be objectionable? ____
_____

Would assisting at a surgical operation bother you? _____
Would you be willing to have a complete medical and dental exam, with a report
filed to this office? _____
What three characteristics best describe you? _____
_____

What short- and long-term goals do you personally have? _____
_____

EDUCATION

Indicate highest grade completed
Elementary   6   7   8
High school   1   2   3   4
College   1   2   3   4   5   6   7   8
Approximate grade point average _____

Age completed: Elementary____ High school_____ College_____ Graduate_____

Approximate number in high school class _____

Approximate class standing _____

Favorite high school subjects _____

Least liked _____

Extracurricular activities _____

_____

Part-time and summer work _____

Class and other offices held _____

Colleges attended and dates attended _____

_____

Major fields _____

Degree(s) and year(s) obtained _____

Extracurricular activities _____

_____

How was your education financed?_____

% expenses you earned? _____

Part-time and summer work in college? _____

_____

MY DENTAL HISTORY

1. Is there someone that you consider as "your dentist?" _____

2. If you were asked to refer someone to a dentist, do you know of one whom
   you would choose?_____ Why? _____

3. If you have changed dentists in the last five years, please indicate:
   ☐ Yes ☐ No
   Circumstances and reasons_____

4. Do you consider your teeth and oral structure to be in:
   Excellent   _____
   Good   _____
   Fair   _____   condition?
   Poor   _____

5. Were your dental services during the past five years thorough and very
   complete? ☐ Yes ☐ No

6. How often have you visited a dentist in the past five years? _____

7. How often did you visit the dentist for preventive examinations?
   Every 3 months_____
   Every 6 months_____

Every year_____
Other_____
If other, please indicate _____
8. What services were performed on these visits? _____
_____

9. Was there any treatment that was suggested, but not performed regarding treatment? _____
10. Was this due to any specific reason? _____
11. My opinion about dentistry is different from other people's because: _____
_____

This is an exact copy of the application form we use in our office. I believe (also hope and pray) that we are violating none of the laws covering fairness and equity in the hiring process. Please feel free to adopt or modify our form for your own use, as you see fit. You may wish to ask your attorney or someone from your state job service to review the form before you use it, to ensure that you haven't inadvertently broken one of the myriad regulations concerning what can and can not be asked of a potential employee.

I have a strong urge to editorialize, possibly to pontificate, on government interference in the hiring process. I guess there is no point to such comments, because the regulations that currently exist won't be changed due to any thoughts of mine. Do be advised that violating these fair employment laws can result in severe penalties. Be certain that whatever form you use is in complete compliance with all state and federal mandates concerning hiring.

The first line of our Personal Record Form states that all the information submitted to us in trust will be held in *strict confidence*. Be sure that all of your staff involved in the hiring process respect and understand this commitment. The confidentiality that is promised is your ethical responsibility to ensure. As with patient confidentiality, this is not a matter to be taken lightly. Be sure that your team is clear that no discussion of the information gathered in the hiring process can ever be allowed outside of the office.

The first paragraph of the form asks the applicant to give you an estimate of what level of compensation they would expect if this position is obtained. The information gained from this query is somewhat difficult to interpret.

If a potential team member lists minimum wage for expected earnings, it could indicate a low self-esteem. It could also mean that she really desires the job as described in the want ad, and money is not a primary motivating factor for her. If she puts down a figure doubling the salary you are able to offer, it is possible you won't be able to afford to hire her. However, over the years I've offered a position to people at a much lower figure than the one they quoted as "earnings expected" and had them accept the position. This figure may give you some insight into the person applying, but use this bit of data carefully and in combination with other information you acquire.

I wouldn't eliminate a candidate just on the basis of this response alone, no matter what earnings estimate they state. If the salary figure quoted is well above what the position available would pay, but you are impressed with the applicant, I would suggest your staff member inform the applicant of the range of possible salaries when she calls to schedule an interview. If this is acceptable, schedule the interview. If it isn't, thank the applicant for their interest and move on in the hiring process. You've saved everyone a lot of time and trouble.

In reviewing the "history of work experience" section of our personal record form, I look carefully for a pattern of too much job mobility. No matter what reasons for switching jobs is given, a person who historically has moved from job to job probably won't be in your office long either. I think you'll often find the reason given for past job movement has something to do with "unfair treatment" in previous jobs. This, at least, is the applicant's perception and/or explanation. My guess is, should you employ them, they will feel unfairly treated by you before long. The two exceptions to this negative perception created for me by job mobility are career advancement opportunities or a geographic move that required a change in employment. I am even suspicious of these moves. Good people tend to find the right employment situation and remain in it.

In addition to stability in past employment, I look for patterns of upward mobility within previous job, both in salary and responsibility. As in the case with my review of the entire form, I analyze this section for *completeness* of answers and *quality of expression*. Many job applicants don't even bother to fully complete all of our admittedly (and deliberately) long form. If they lack the commitment to completely fill out an application, how well do you believe they will perform if given the job? I also like to study the applicant's use of language in filling out the application. I believe a form that could be answered with *yes* or *no* responses would greatly reduce my ability to see into the mind of an applicant.

Be certain when you arrive at the point in your hiring process that involves reference checks that you are cognizant of any employers the applicant has asked you on the application *not* to contact. If it was a previous employer the applicant doesn't want contacted, I'd like to know why we shouldn't communicate with them. I would listen very carefully to the candidate's explanation. Is there a chance that something occurred on that job that our potential team member doesn't want us to know? However, never risk an applicant's current job by contacting the employer without permission. Sometimes the employer is aware of the applicant's plans to leave their employ and will be an excellent source of information. Be very certain this is the case before contacting them. I would hate to be responsible, legally or morally, for the dismissal of a job applicant due to an unauthorized inquiry from my staff.

Under the "Activities and Interests" section of the form, we again ask what starting salary they would expect if selected for the position. Very often the figure listed here varies from the one recorded on the first page of the application. You may wish to question this inconsistency. You will see a good number of questions duplicated in the different parts of our hiring process. This is not carelessness or error on our part. I am always amazed at the different answers given to the same question, asked at different times and places in our employment routine. Sometimes these variations may just indicate the applicant has had time to consider the matter more carefully. Other times it will reveal a tendency to be "creative" with the truth.

As we mentioned earlier when discussing the phone interview, hobbies and activities that our applicant participates in can give us some very useful information.

Questions such as, "What are your plans for the future?" and "Why do you work?" help us identify values and goals of the applicants, as well as display their ability to express themselves.

Under "Physical Data," I wish to identify smokers and be sure all candidates are physically able to perform the job. Many years ago I hired a chairside that couldn't stand to watch us give local anesthetic. She had a three-day career in our office. (By the end of three days she had backed so far away from the treatment areas that she was out in the street!) Better for the both of us if we had identified her distress at any surgical procedure before employing her.

We ask all applicants if they are "willing to have a complete medical and dental exam." We won't require it, but if the answer is *no*, I want an explanation. A friend of mine once hired a chairside with early multiple sclerosis. It was a sad situation for everyone involved when they all realized she wasn't capable of doing the job.

The questions on personal goals and a self-description of the applicant again give you a chance to examine values and writing ability. As you can see, I like to scatter the questions that provide me with information about the person, and not just their factual history, throughout the form. I believe this provides more insight than lumping all similar questions in one area.

Under the education section of the application, I want to see what level of training and/or formal education they have achieved, of course. I enjoy the company of intelligent and well-educated people, and this information helps me to identify them. (Note that I didn't say I was one, I just said that I enjoy the company of well-educated people.) I'm also interested in their work ethic. A detailed account of summer jobs and methods used in helping to pay for college expenses often illustrates the type of work ethic I admire in a fellow employee.

We have touched on my feeling about the critical importance of the dental history as an indicator for potential success as an employee in my office. Please forgive my redundancy, but I would give this section of the application your most careful evaluation. I have had applicants that were excellent in every area we considered except their dental values. I have hired them in spite of this shortcoming and have been sorry every time. I think a lot of you will minimize the importance of this factor as a predictor of employment success (as I did). I'm pretty sure you'll regret it if you do.

At this point, we have all the factual data we will gather, and I have to review the information obtained during the process and select people I will be personally interviewing. I lean heavily on my staff evaluations, both on the phone interview and their observations of potential team members as applications were being filled out in our office reception area. I have in the past ignored their input and scheduled an interview with an applicant that "looks good on paper," but whom my staff had rated poorly. Usually I know the person isn't right for the job two minutes after we begin talking. We have wasted not only my time and the applicant's, but the time and talent of the team member whose judgment we have ignored.

After a through review of all the data we have collected, I usually select from six to eight people to interview. I set aside one hour to spend with each candidate. We try to schedule everyone within the time frame of a few days if possible. I tend to forget some details of our discussion, no matter how carefully I take notes, if too long a time passes between the first and last interview. The impressions made by the most recently interviewed applicants are so much stronger than those made by earlier candidates that the entire interview process is biased. The choice to do all the interviews as closely together as possible often means an entire day will be devoted to the task. Staff members are so critical to the success of any practice that a day devoted to nothing but interviews is a small price to pay considering the value to be gained.

I have been forced by the limited availability of a candidate to conduct interviews in the evening after work. I think this is unfair both to the interviewer and to the applicant because neither of you is at your best. I interview at the end of a working day only if no other physical possibility for us to meet exists.

The personal interview is a critical step in the hiring process. Everything possible must be done to maximize its effectiveness. Please remember, dentists aren't trained to interview prospective employees, and most of us are probably only fair (at best) in the subtle art of interviewing. Knowing this, we must do everything possible to ensure ourselves of the best possible chance to gain the most valuable and least-biased information possible from the interview.

Before I greet each applicant, I will have again reviewed *all* the forms that have been filled out to date and completed what parts of the summary form (contained later in this chapter) I could, based on the information that we have gathered prior to the interview. I will make a written list of any special concerns or questions I want to ask a particular candidate. When I am confident my preparation for this interview is complete, I will go to our reception room and personally greet the person waiting for me there.

I always shake hands and introduce myself to the interviewee. The degree of "cold and clammy" I find in the grip, tells me the degree of apprehension that exists. This apprehension is my enemy, as it can hide the best qualities of some excellent individuals. I don't wish to hire someone who is skilled at the art of interviewing. Thus my concern is not with their skills during the interview process, but with their potential as a team member. I want all applicants at their best during this interview. It is a major responsibility of the interviewer to allow whatever time is needed to create an environment where the applicant can relax and be at their best. This is similar to the beginning of all new patient interviews, also done in my private office. A relaxed, pleasant, informal atmosphere is most conducive to the outcome we desire in both new patient and job applicant interviews.

I ask the candidate to be seated in my office. We will not be disturbed for any reason during this interview. I begin by thanking them for making the effort to apply and for their interest in our office. I truly am grateful. Often I compliment them on their appearance, and we chat a few minutes on whatever neutral topic seems appropriate, from weather to mutual friends and interests. I already know a lot about them from reviewing our forms, so finding an interesting topic to begin our discussion is simple. My staff has checked our computer, and if the applicant has been in our office as a patient, I have their dental records available. It's unfortunate to begin an interview by introducing yourself to an existing patient as though she were a stranger.

Once I sense by their tone and by their body language that they have relaxed, I begin the formal interview. I start by apologizing. I explain that I don't interview often, and that due to my deficiencies as an interviewer, I will ask them the same series of "patterned" questions that I ask each applicant. I add that I feel asking each person the identical questions gives a more equitable outcome to the interview process. I also add that I will take some notes during their responses, and please don't be distracted by my scribbling.

I assure the interviewee the questions I will ask have no right or wrong answer, but are simply intended to help me get to know them. I encourage them to ask me questions at any time. We then proceed to the patterned interview.

I tend to talk too much. This is *always* a mistake, but it is a deadly sin in an interview. (My M.D. brother Jim recently informed me that: (1) You never lose weight eating, and (2) you never learn anything by talking. Both bits of advice seem accurate, but I have no idea why he happened to share this wealth of the obvious with me!) The patterned-question format helps limit my tendency to wax, if not elegant, at least lengthy. I used to spend a lot of time explaining the job details during the interview. That got tedious, even for a "talker." I hand the Job Benefit Description to the interviewee when they first ask a question about working conditions. I give them a minute to peruse this document, and I answer any questions they have about it. Not only does the job description form save time, but in case there exists a misunderstanding concerning benefits at a later date, we have this standard document we reviewed together to refer back to.

When we complete the hiring process, we require each new staff member to read our office policy manual and sign a statement saying that she understands its content. This manual contains in much greater detail all the information concerning employment conditions and regulations in our office. The brief job description is simply a "shorthand" version, to save our precious interview time.

JOB BENEFIT DESCRIPTION

Three-month probationary period before benefits become effective. Starting salary $5 to $8 an hour depending on the level of previous experience.

Six paid holidays a year.

One week paid vacation after one year of employment.
Two weeks paid vacation after two years of employment.
Health bonus—½ day paid sick leave per month. If employees do not use their sick day, they receive this benefit in salary.

All uniforms purchased by office.

Workman's Compensation Insurance.

Continuing education—all expenses paid and salary paid on normal working days.

All dental work free except for lab bills. Twenty-five percent off for family members.

Retirement plan.

PATTERNED PERSONAL INTERVIEW

1. What are three things you do to promote your good health? _____
   _____

2. What do you do to promote your own dental health? _____
   _____

3. What quality do you value most in other people? _____
   _____

4. What kind of persons do you prefer to work with? _____
   _____

5. What is most important to you in a job? _____
   What do you care least about in a job? _____

6. What job do you wish to have in five years? _____

7. How do you react when you are asked to work overtime? _____
   _____

8. What additional training do you feel you need to realize your career goals?
   _____

9. Would you rather be assigned a task and be responsible for it or do you
   prefer to work with someone else at all times? _____
   Why? _____

10. What situations have you found most stressful on the job? _____
    _____

    What techniques have you found to manage these stresses? _____
    _____

11. What words do other people use to describe you? _____

12. If you have a variety of tasks which you need to accomplish in a given
    period of time, what approach do you take? _____
    _____

13. How do you react when treated unfairly in an every day situation? _____
    _____

14. How do you feel about taking on additional responsibility? _____
    _____

15. What impression do you think you create with other people? _____
    _____

16. What plans do you have for your own personal improvement? _____
    _____

17. Of what three accomplishments are you most proud? _____
    _____

18. How have your past job experiences prepared you for this position? _____

_____

19. What is your interpretation of "success"? _____

_____

20. If you could structure the perfect job for yourself, what would you do and why? _____

I don't believe I've ever asked all the questions on this form to any one applicant. The form functions as a guide to lead the conversation. The point isn't to fill out this form, but to determine if the individual I'm currently interviewing will become a member of our team. I have some specific questions prepared especially for this individual based on the application information we have previously gathered. Usually I will make these queries after the patterned interview is completed, when the maximum understanding between us has been established.

I believe by now, dear reader, you possess enough information on our hiring system to evaluate the style and purpose of the patterned-interview questions. They are all open-ended questions that encourage the applicant to speak. The aim of each question is more to identify values than to establish facts. As this discussion proceeds I evaluate the applicant for an overall impression too. Is she poised? How is her grammar? Do you notice a sense of humor present? *Is this someone you would enjoy working with?*

The patterned questions begin by requesting relatively easy, factual information and then grow more abstract. You will wish to develop your own interview questions based on the values your team has identified. That is how it should be. My emphasis here is not to discuss the particular questions of our form, but to establish the benefits of a patterned interview format.

We end the interview promptly at the scheduled time. I ask if there are any questions our applicant has that I may answer. When I have responded to her questions, I thank our candidate again for her time, and promise to notify her as soon as we have reached a hiring decision. I think immediate notification of the outcome of the hiring process is the least you owe these people for the time they have invested with you. This promise of notification also saves us time by preventing each candidate from calling the office and "quizzing" the staff about how close to reaching a final decision we are.

Over the years a number of new patient families have come from people we interviewed and didn't hire. Please remember that the hiring process represents your office as much as every other function your team performs. These applicants are judging you and your staff, even as you evaluate them. That judgment will be carried to the community. As always, we wish the impression our office leaves with people to be a positive one.

As soon as my office door has closed behind the applicant, I begin to fill out our Summary Form. I allow myself 10 minutes of the allotted hour interview period for this task and for reviewing the information for the next interview. I have a lot of the summary form already completed from information gathered before the interview, but I want to record pertinent facts about the interview while it is completely fresh in my mind, and not after six more interviews have taken place. The information condensed on our summary form will be critical in helping me reach a final hiring decision.

SUMMARY FORMS

Name: _____ Age:_____

Application letter: _____

Appearance and voice: _____

Work history (skills and experience): _____

_____

Motivation to work; aims in life; achievement of goals: _____

_____

Health: _____Chronic disease, days missed last year:_____

Education: _____

Dental history: _____

Family background: Marriage, parents and siblings, children, support for working: _____

Social background: activities enjoyed, leadership: _____

_____

Test scores: _____

Reference check: _____

Comments: _____

_____

Job strengths and weaknesses: _____

Recommendations: _____

When the interviewing is completed, I sit down with a hot cup of coffee, and once again truncate our list of possible candidates. Usually by this point in the process we will have from two to four candidates still under consideration. Sometimes I have one candidate that seems clearly superior to all the other applicants. If that is so, I will proceed to our final hiring steps with her alone involved. If in these final steps a question of her suitability arises, I will go back and review the information on our other finalists.

More frequently there will be two or three fairly equal applicants. If that is the case, all of them will remain involved in the final steps of our hiring process.

The next step in our selection process is to check references on each remaining candidate. The reference checks are *critical.* They are also difficult and tricky to do. They are performed by the same senior staff member who did the phone interviews. Often our best information comes from fellow workers at a previous job. We seldom contact the references listed by the candidate, on the theory that anyone can find three people who like them. We use these sources only if we aren't allowed access to previous places of employment. We try to get *three* completed reference checks on each applicant still under consideration.

Always check references. It can save you from embezzlement and many other potential headaches, as well as greatly add to the information you possess on each applicant. Frequently a very strong or a very weak reference will sway the final hiring decision.

In our office, if a reference check is requested by a potential employer of a past member of our team, we give out only the dates of employment of the former staff person and their beginning and ending compensation. That is it! To do more puts you at risk of potential litigation. All of my staff are carefully instructed in this regard, because even if the call they get concerning references on a former employee is received at their home, I am legally responsible for their responses. Please call the employment department of any industry around you and ask for information about former employees. Dates of employment and beginning and final salary is all the information you will be given. If you decide to help a dentist buddy and give out more information (which I have done), at least be aware that you are opening yourself to potential legal action.

Good news! Most dentists are too uninformed to know this and will just blabber away about a previous employee. One told me he wouldn't touch the b—— with a ten-foot pole. I'd guess he risked his life savings with that comment. Hope he enjoyed it. At any rate, with a little persistence and ingenuity, you can still usually get this vital reference check information. Just be dead certain your staff isn't giving it out.

REFERENCE CHECK

"I would appreciate your helping me to obtain information on _____ _____ who is applying for a position with us. Do you remember her?"

1. When did she work for you? from_____ to _____
2. She lists her salary as_____. Is that correct?
3. What kind of work did she do? _____
4. Is she a good worker? _____
5. Does she get along well with others? _____
6. What do you think of her? _____
7. What were her strong points? _____
8. What were her weak points? _____
9. Why did she leave?_____
10. Did she have any problems that interfered with her work? Specify: _____
    _____
11. Would you rehire her?_____ If not, why? _____
12. Is there anything else you would like to tell us about her?_____
    Comments? _____

The key question in any reference check: *Would you hire her again?* If they wouldn't, after working with her, do you want to employ her? Review the information you have obtained from your reference checks carefully for inconsistencies with what your applicant has told you. There could exist differences in perceptions concerning some information. Be aware there may also be some outright lies discovered. A lie on a factual matter, such as salary level or date of employment, would most likely eliminate that applicant as a candidate.

I believe this final step in our hiring process is critical too. We now invite the remaining applicant or applicants to work for one-half day (with pay) in our office, and then to go to lunch at the office's expense with all staff members of her future department. You, doctor, are not invited.

In the half day spent working in our office, the candidate may find this isn't the place for her. Much better to find out now than three months from now, when you get to practice the hiring process all over again! Your staff will let her do some simple tasks during this half day and see if she performs them well, but the main thing we wish to observe is *attitude*. This is not a part of job training, but the last step in candidate evaluation.

The "free lunch" (Remember, there is no free lunch. Not here or anywhere else.) is the last part of the *hiring process*, but the applicant doesn't know that. The *boss* isn't there, and often the candidate will let her hair down, having lunch with "just the girls." Twice I have decided not to hire people based on the results of some very candid information obtained by my trained staff at these lunches.

This final staff involvement provides us with one more source of information, but its value is far greater than that. If the candidate's future co-workers say "hire her," *they have made a commitment to her success.* They will work harder to support her, because she is *their choice* for the position. I suppose there are many ways to get the staff to support a new staff member. Such support is vital if the new member of your team has any hope of being successful. If she is resented and not helped by existing staff, she will fail. Lunch and a half-day's salary is a small price to pay for this commitment.

The next step is for the senior member of the department to call and "hire" her new team member. Our senior member makes the actual job offer, because she made the hiring decision, along with her fellow department staff, remember? All the details of the job are discussed, and a date to begin employment is agreed upon. The department can now finalize their plans for training this new associate. A definite schedule that lists what tasks will be taught, who will teach each separate skill, and when that training will occur, will be given to our new staff member as soon as she reports for duty.

With our new team member on board, it's time to send the candidates we interviewed but didn't hire "sorry" letters. Be certain before sending these notifications that the person you offered the job has accepted and is eager to begin. These letters are often accompanied by flowers and a personal note of thanks to the one or two applicants who came the closest to being hired. Remember, even with all the care and effort involved in our hiring system, there is no guarantee that the person you select will work out. You may very well find yourself offering a position to one of these people you are now rejecting, possibly in the near future. You may also be performing a new-patient examination of her soon. In short, you have good reasons to maintain as positive a relationship as possible with the people you interviewed.

REJECTION LETTER

Dear

I am very sorry to inform you that you were not selected to fill our current staff vacancy. We had a large number of qualified people apply and only one position to fill. I want to thank you for your time and effort and wish you the best of luck in finding the job you desire and deserve. It was a pleasure meeting with you.

Sincerely,

John A. Wilde and Staff

Is this hiring process a lot of work? You bet! Can you take a shortcut and pick and choose the steps you like? I guess. It all depends on your *values*. How important is the best possible staff to you? Lots of dentists don't have the time for this. Oh, they would if they made as much money as I do. But if they continue to hire unsuitable staff members, do you think they will ever achieve financial success? I hope you get the point. Hiring the right staff is a crucial part of team building. I promise, you *cannot* spend too much in time or money on any facet of this team-building task.

Now that you have all the information necessary to hire an outstanding team, ask yourself these questions:

1. Will this outstanding individual who so closely mirrors our office values work for the lowest possible benefit and salary package?

2. Will she accept employment in a run-down and poorly appearing physical facility?

Consistency and values are again the keys. The staff, the office they work in, the way they are treated, and the materials and equipment used must consistently reflect your beliefs. *You will not keep great people in a mediocre office*. Don't waste your time trying to hire the best unless you are committed to being the best. Not the Superman of dentists, but a dentist completely committed to being the best you can be. Use this system to find and hire winners. Then enjoy the success that your efforts have created.

CHAPTER 10

OFFICE IDENTITY

Many and varied are the roads that can lead to success in dentistry. None of these paths are right or wrong in any absolute sense. However, there does exist one best path for each of us. By now, you should be well on your way to discovering the "path with meaning" that exists for you. Through the process of self-discovery and value clarification you are pursuing, as well as with the staff meeting, communication exercises, and team-building steps that are being activated in your office, a clear personal and office identity will begin to slowly but surely emerge.

To better help you find and follow your path, I want to share with you an image of how some other successful dental paths look by examining the stories of three dental offices. All three practices are highly successful. All exemplify the vision of three very deliberate, foresighted leaders. Despite these similarities, the three offices could hardly be more different from each other in their approach to uncommon success in dentistry.

Get a fresh cup of coffee and relax. It's fun to read stories, especially true ones. But, as you enjoy this narrated journey, be searching for a clearer picture of *your* identity. None of these offices will be identical to yours. You may wish to incorporate a few of the behaviors described here for your own use; that is fine. But you must weave those tidbits into a fabric that is uniquely and individually yours. To do so you must first deeply understand *who you are*. Once you obtain that awareness, you can accept and incorporate into your practice the ideas presented here that are truly consistent with your identity and not just copy some concepts you believe sound good.

On to our story.

My favorite stories have a bad guy, but in this tale there exists only three good guys. In addition to the story's lack of a villain, this tale is also made different by this unusual circumstance: nobody loses! In fact, all three protagonists win, and they win big in their own uniquely individual ways. That fact makes this a happy story, but let me hasten to assure you, it does have a moral!

Here we have a tale of three unique habitats, constructed most deliberately by leaders with strong visions. Coincidentally, all of the entities we will observe are dental offices. Don't let that accident limit your own search for experiences. I have learned much from studying the disciplines of education, psychology, business, and religion (to name but a few). All these fields contain information of great value that can be used to edify, guide, and stimulate us in our dental futures. Use every resource you can find to assist you in your journey. It is only for the sake of this example that we will limit ourselves to stories of dental success.

Protagonist A practices dentistry in a Midwestern community of 45,000. I'll give you a clue to his identity: he is a past clinical director of the Pankey Institute. (For the few of you who are unaware, the Pankey Institute is a private continuing-education facility in Florida. They conduct week-long courses in dental excellence for practicing dentists. I believe it fair to say that the Pankey Institute attempts to teach excellence in life as well as dentistry.) A number of years ago our hero discontinued his work at the institute to return to his home town and begin a private practice. He had practiced there before joining the people at Pankey full time.

His physical plant is beautiful. The door going into his office sets the tone. I wish I had the skills to describe that door the way I'd like to: the beauty of the wood and the ornate lights on either side of the door that frame it. Before you may enter his office, you must physically confront this door. The appearance of that door alone speaks volumes. If asked to describe those who inhabited the space behind this portal, most people would guess that the inhabitants stand for substance, quality, beauty, and function. They would be correct.

When you enter the reception room (no one would be so crass as to describe this as a waiting room), you will perceive that your assumptions arrived at by analyzing the door's exterior were correct. Inside is a scene of quiet beauty. The plants, carpet, and furnishings (even the subject matter of the magazines) are obviously carefully selected. All repeat the same message as the door. They undeniably identify those who dwell within.

I once heard my friend asked if he wasn't afraid that the beautiful carpet and furnishings would be damaged by thoughtless or clumsy patients. He said that people aren't careless in such an environment. The behavior of the people who enter the room conforms to the physical surroundings they find themselves in. I guess you could see the same thing at a church or some other place of solemn gatherings. The physical presence controls the behavior of the people in that space without a word needing to be said.

The dental equipment and furnishings that make up the rest of the office are similarly tasteful, of obvious beauty and quality. The paintings, plants, and decorations all reflect deliberate care, taste, and purpose in their selection.

As soon as you have entered the reception area, you will be greeted by the receptionist. The staff of three are attractive people in their thirties and forties. Your immediate impression would be of the warmth of the smile and the genuineness of the welcome offered. You would be greeted by name, I assure you. The doctor has told me a number of times that the sweetest sound any person ever hears is the sound of their own name.

You would probably be one of five or six patients scheduled that day. The doctor does TMJ and reconstructive work almost exclusively. Let's assume you're a new patient arriving for an examination. The medical forms and other questions you expect to be asked to fill out with the conventional pen and clipboard to support your efforts would instead be completed by the receptionist in an interview format, thus enhancing the personal quality of the service. When the forms are completed and have been explained and discussed, the examination would begin.

The doctor will enter the room, shake your hand, and introduce himself by his name, not his title. "Hi, Sue. I'm Fred. It's a real pleasure to welcome you to our office." He will be dressed casually, *sans* tie. (It is probably a coincidence, but none of the winning doctors in the three offices we'll discuss wear a tie. Does this mean they have congenitally warm necks?)

One of the doctors in our office recently asked that he always be addressed as "doctor" in the presence of patients in the name of "professionalism." How you feel about this tells a lot about your self-image and philosophy. Think it over. No, I'm not going to explain it to you.

The time allotted for this dental examination is 60 minutes. I used to wonder what they did during a 60-minute dental examination. The answer is: mostly talk. But that isn't really correct. From the doctor's standpoint at least, what is done most is listening! I believe Dr. Omar Reed tells his audience, "If you must speak during this patient interview, *ask a question!*" The impression you want to make is not how erudite you are, but how much you care about the other person involved in the conversation. Do you wish to know how to give every patient you see the impression that you really care about them? It's simple. You just really do care.

I'm not as familiar with the financial situation of this office as I am with that of the other two practices in our story. I do know a TMJ splint is inserted at an investment (not an expense or cost. The words we use do have meaning to patients) of over $700, and that a crown fee exceeds $1,000 (yes, that is per unit). How do you feel about that?

I used to feel that my fees were a direct extension of myself, that if a patient refused care or left the office, he refused and left *me*. I don't feel that way any more, but it took a lot of cogitation on the delicate but crucial issue of money to clarify my thoughts. Have you thought deeply about fees? Are you uncomfortable quoting them to your patients? These feelings won't go away until you clarify your own values about money and the fees you charge.

In the three offices we are touring I believe the crown fees to range from roughly $300 to $500 to $1,000. If there are three such widely varying fees, (in effect three answers to the same question, "How much for a cap, Doc?") that means two of them must be wrong— correct? No, I'm not going to explain it to you.

People come to any office aware of the style of dentistry being practiced within. I doubt this office gets a lot of "yellow page" or "shopper" type patients. Very few individuals choose this quality of care, yet I believe this office to be busier than it wishes to be. They have added an associate dentist in the last few years, but the owner of the practice sees patients about the same 100 days I do. (No, this sure isn't my office, but we do have a nice front door.) Stop for a second now, and imagine for yourself what the vision of this office would be.

Let's move on to the dwelling place of our second dentist hero. (Doesn't the phrase "dentist hero" sound nice? And why not? We *are* deserving.) This practice is located in another Midwestern town of about 100,000 souls. It is a three-doctor practice, located in a free-standing, three-story building that previously had been a travel agency. The owner began his career as a very successful pedodontist, then retired from dentistry for five years. Fifteen years ago, at the age of 47, he started his career over again as a general dentist.

The door to this office is nondescript, or at least in my many visits I haven't noticed it. Maybe the large, lighted sign in front and the giant toothbrush that helps announce the practice too fully capture my attention. When you do open that door, you'll be greeted by a real buzz of activity. There is a staff of 36 waiting to serve you. There are five hygienists and a full laboratory with three technicians on the premises. There is a dress code here. All staff (including doctors) wear designer jeans. Over 200 new patients are seen each month, many of them on some type of welfare or entitlement program. I believe the last figure I heard for monthly production was $185,000. I'm sure it's higher today.

The vision in this office is one of quickness and efficiency. This is not the abode of the 60-minute new-patient interview. The phone is always answered quickly, and the voice you hear is always pleasant. The staff is young, usually cute, and the faces seem to change often. All of them are busy. They work in an atmosphere of pleasantness, but every patient must be aware of the efficiency and promptness of all those who toil within.

This office does a lot of excellent and creatively unique marketing. Since a great deal of their care is denture work, much of their marketing effort is pitched to the geriatric patient. They sponsor the local time and temperature phone line in their community, which gives out, along with the requested information, a short commercial for their office.

On Thanksgiving Day this doctor prepares and serves, at his personal expense, a full Thanksgiving dinner to all who choose to come and partake. This annual event has been going on for years. It is a complete dining experience, including live music and roses to be taken home by the guests. Last year 4,000 people attended, served by dozens of volunteers from the community. The short message given by the host doctor at the dinner said that at this time of year especially, we all need to be together, and that the only ticket needed for next year's dinner was to return and bring a friend.

The coverage of the event by the local paper and TV stations is extensive. Volunteers to help serve the food and to deliver it to shut-ins have to be turned away, because more volunteer to help than can be used. I present this as one example of extraordinary marketing and of the unusual spirit of caring for others embodied in this office and in this event.

The owner of this office has written three dental books, innumerable dental articles, newspaper columns, and an on-going monthly column for a free geriatric newsletter. He also speaks at dental meetings and is an expert on dental computers. Here is another coincidence: while none of the doctors wear ties, all have extensive computer systems. One doctor writes a computer column in a dental magazine; another owns a Computer Land store.

Note in all these details the focus. The staff is dressed to be "just folks." The emphasis is on a lot of people paying a moderate fee for friendly, quality care. This is a volume practice, where the owner himself is chairside more than 200 days a year and loves it. Organization, efficiency, the ability to treat many people in a short time, and providing the treatment without sacrificing the importance of the individual: these are themes of this practice. How does this compare in your mind with our first office? Which is you? How would your feelings about fees influence either of these situations?

Our third office is a small group practice of three dentists in a town of 13,000. The decor is pleasant, but certainly not opulent. The staff wear matching uniforms, as most teams in any form of endeavor do. Most of the staff members have been in the practice for many years and are old friends to the patients.

The atmosphere is pleasant, friendly, and informal. Patients are addressed by their first names, and staff members wear name tags with their first names scripted to help identify them as individuals to the patients, not just interchangeable nonentities. Staff people will spend time just talking to patients. Such "meaningless" chatter is encouraged.

Notes in green pen concerning personal happenings in the patients'" lives (birthdays, anniversaries, vacations, as well as illness, loss of a loved one, etc.) are recorded in the records to be recalled at future visits, so patients feel they are recognized and appreciated as individuals. Taking the time to note these personal events in green pen is a manifestation of caring. When these personal details are recalled by the staff at the next visit, the patient is made aware of your regard for them as a person, not just a patient. Here is a marketing procedure that costs you nothing to implement, and thus its return is infinite!

The reception room looks a lot like a middle-class family's living room, but not much like a dental reception area. No dental literature is on display, and there is a picture of the owner's family on the wall. You'd notice he has four children. It's a relief if you are a parent trusting him with your children's dental care to know the doctor has young kids too.

The doctor is casually dressed here also and was even before the OSHA uniform code was in effect. He also introduces himself by his name, *sans* doctor. The new patient exam lasts 30 minutes, but also involves a lot of listening. Production in this office is about $60,000 per month, and collections are close to 100%. Overhead is carefully controlled, and all staff members are very aware of their unique duties as members of the team. The fees are a little above the norm for this area.

What identifies this office is its focus on the middle-class family, and on friendly, but extremely efficient, care. A wide range of procedures from TMJ to orthopedics is offered. Evening and Saturday hours are available. The team is quick and professional, yet unfailingly friendly. Care is both gentle and personal for each and every patient treated.

Do you see the point of this journey? The first office we visited was very successful! Its clientele were mostly prominent and wealthy individuals who desired the best in dental care and who would and could pay to receive it.

The second office was very successful! It focused on quick, efficient care at lower fees for a mostly blue-collar clientele. These were patients with little spare time, so night and evening hours were available. Their clients were not, for the most part, wealthy, yet they wanted quality care. They received good, basic, affordable dental treatment in an atmosphere that was friendly, professional, and efficient.

The third office was very successful! It was a family-oriented practice. They saw a little of both wealthy and indigent, but the backbone of the office was treating families with children. The reception room decor was nice, but also featured a separate play area for the kids who would be coming along for dental care. No fine art or crystal is on display.

As I said earlier, these offices are all unique, yet they are all winners. One treats seven patients a day, another 35, and a third sees 100 or more. One charges fees that are high by any standard and does complex state-of-the-art dental care.

Our second office has fees that are low and care that is basic.

The third office falls in the center of this continuum. To my eye these offices are as diverse as it is possible to imagine. (I assure you, these are *real* dental practices, not conjured up to make my point.)

So different, and yet all so successful. Do you know why? *It is the clarity of values and vision.* It doesn't matter that the visions are so diverse. What matters (and the reason behind the success of each) is the precise nature of the vision and the singlemindedness displayed in its pursuit. Each facet of the office—its appearance, the attitude of the staff, the tone of the office, the fee scale, the style of the patient interaction— all focus on one clearly defined objective. Every person employed in each of the three offices knows precisely what his/her team and personal objectives are.

This is the touchstone for your success. First, you must identify exactly who you are and what you believe. Once this is clearly established, then every decision you make in your practice and your life must be consistent with this image. Your lamp shades and your toilet fixtures must match this self-view.

Any action or physical presence that isn't consistent, no matter how good the reason for its being there (your mom gave it to you; it was on sale for half off), blurs your vision's focus and strikes a dissident cord.

Get another cup of coffee, if you choose. Then sit down with a blank piece of paper and describe your office. Discuss this with your team, or better yet, have them do a similar exercise; then compare notes. This exercise in defining who you are and what you wish to become could be the first step on your team's journey to success.

CHAPTER 11

THE SECRET TO THE SUCCESSFUL IMPLEMENTATION OF NEW IDEAS

(And the Explanation of Why These Ideas Sometimes Fail)

This chapter is based on an article I wrote, published by *Dental Economics* magazine in the February 1993 issue. A lot of the ideas in it are somewhat similar to the philosophy discussions of earlier chapters. Remember, a leader's task is to get a vision and repeat it. I've included the article for three reasons:

1. I know this is shallow, but I like this pretentious, overdone style. Call it my flowery period. Anyway, one chapter won't hurt you.

2. Some of the concepts (for example, the main discussion of why ideas succeed or fail in your office and life) are a new twist to our familiar theme of clarifying values and setting goals.

3. I like some of the illustrations and examples in this article. These are very pragmatic examples of our philosophy in action. I hope these additional illustrations will help you to understand more completely the concepts we discussed earlier.

I fully understand that most of you clipped this article and saved it. (I assume some of you memorized it and thus had no need to clip it.) At least with it included in this book you'll know where to find it!

Have you ever gone to a dental meeting and heard a *great idea?* An idea so incredible that you carefully wrap it and lovingly transport it back to your office. At the next staff meeting, with trembling hands, The Idea is gently unveiled, usually to the ohhhs and ahhhs customarily accorded a newborn. With shivers of anticipation, the perfect action plan to implement The Idea is sculpted. The proper commitments are made by appropriate people, and The Idea is launched! Usually it's a few weeks, sometimes a few months, before you realize that *we are no longer doing it!*

For years I lived with this frustration: to be cursed with a staff somehow incapable of the detection and follow-through of genius. But sometimes they could and did follow through. Some of the ideas took root and became a permanent part of our office life. So what twists of chance choose life or death for these worthy concepts? Was it merely the capricious whims of a sometimes fickle fate, or the collective tides of our office biorhythm that controlled the success or failure of these thoughts?

There was indeed a dark force that sabotaged my "best laid plans." Over the years, I searched for the key to this seemingly random presence that controlled the fate of our new ideas and thus controlled the very ability of our office to grow and prosper. As the years passed, I met this secret enemy, and just as Pogo has so sagely predicted, the enemy was *me.* Let me elucidate further the discovery and eventual demise of this pernicious influence that so affected the fate of myself, my staff, and the collective well-being of our office.

Examples of the successfully adopted Great Ideas over the years are legion: full-mouth surveys, and later panorexes replaced the sporadic bite wings of earlier years. Blood-pressure measurement on each patient, reviewing medical histories at every visit, as well as an insistence that our office be timely, that patients were seldom forced to wait. These and many similar ideas over the years became the foundation of our office's success and were permanently adopted by our staff.

But the failed and discarded ideas, stillborn even as we speak: to have patients make a return visit for the polishing of amalgam restorations. To ask patients in terms polished to the sheen of perfection by role playing to refer their friends and family to our care. These and many more fill the tomb of Great Ideas not to be.

How could my staff, so loyal and so wise, not have helped these concepts to fruition? Surely these ideas were worthy and would have proven an asset to our office.

The answer was simple, if not pleasant. The terrible flaw that doomed these ideas was me! Or perhaps more correctly, my personal level of commitment and belief in a particular concept. This was the critical factor that either assured the success of these inspirations or lead to their eventual failure. You see, I never did like to polish amalgams, and my staff doing them (if truth be known) kept them from more productive and possibly profitable endeavors while tying up needed and valuable operatory space. As long as we're being candid, I never felt very comfortable asking people to refer their friends and family to our office. I think it's a good, simple, and honest plan. Lord knows, I've heard and read it recommended often enough. I just never felt at ease requesting it! But why didn't my staff support me here? We held staff meeting after staff meeting to discuss it, and even developed a bonus plan based on new patients seen in the office, but still that critical request for referrals was seldom made.

The problem was congruency, (or lack of same) on my part. Who was it spoke the fateful words, "What you do speaks so loudly that I can not hear what you say"? Like it or not, by some form of osmosis my staff discerned a certain level of discomfort that existed within me. Somehow these fine ideas didn't sit right with my own personal values, and just as I couldn't support them verbally, I also didn't support them at some deeper, internal level. Despite all my elegant words and efforts, my subconscious lack of commitment meant the fledgling concepts were doomed to failure.

Were these ideas evil? Were these concepts fated to fail, poorly developed, or badly conceived? No, they simply were not consistent with my own personal values, the internal or true being that is the real me.

So what does the loss of these abandoned ideas ultimately mean? A little time and energy is wasted. No big deal, and no harm done, right? I'm not too sure. Think about how you feel when you sense, or outright know, a person's actions vary from his or her true beliefs. At best it makes you question, at worst it leads to a loss of trust, both in that individual, and their further proclamations. Other ideas and statements now must be evaluated and carefully analyzed, not simply taken on faith.

I would further like to submit that this evaluative process is universal, that this same premise will hold as true for your one-year-old or your dog. Namely, that when you see or sense inconsistency between a person's words and deeds, the price paid includes a weakening in the bonds of trust. To me, this is a very dear price to pay, indeed!

Now, if this weakening of trust, be it with staff, patients, or the afore-mentioned canine, is a bill you don't wish to pay, how can it be avoided?

Well, I have good news and bad. The bad news: while you can avoid this inconsistency between your values and actions, it's done by an alchemy both difficult and imprecise. The good news: this process pays dividends beyond the most greedy banker's wildest dreams.

The solution is to become *consciously* aware of your values. This is the insurance needed so you won't unwittingly betray the trust of those near and/or dear to you. The values you may have inadvertently violated are there. They already exist in you. The Gordian knot: to clearly identify them and thus avoid the debt that must be paid when your true values are betrayed.

I've read a lot over the years about value clarification. Many people more talented than I have tried to codify exact techniques to accomplish this critical and endless task, so vital to a meaningful life. If a foolproof method has been discovered, it has eluded my detection. However, the *process* of value clarification seems to me to be simply a matter of deliberately becoming aware of your feelings. It means a quiet place, perhaps a fresh cup of coffee, and a blank piece of paper.

With this armor in place, one can sit in the silence of his or her own thoughts and search for the Grail: a clear idea of what he or she truly believes. The critical question: do I believe in this idea enough to give it *my full support!* Half support has no place in your true values. Neither does supporting a project enough to ask others to do the labor involved for you. Jesus said that you must be hot or cold. If you are lukewarm, He will spit you out of his mouth. Who among us is desirous of any more saliva? If you expect a new concept to be adopted by your team, you must be certain that the idea is 100% consistent with your own personal values before you bring the topic up.

There exists in this search a great risk: it is often painful to find out what your values truly are. I mean, isn't everyone supposed to be in favor of a clean house? What will your mom think if she finds out that, deep down, a clean house is not something you're really committed to? But take heart. All the people around you: staff, family, and even mom, already know that which you truly esteem. Despite these insights into your character, they're still there for you. No one judges us as hard as we judge ourselves. Don't allow a fear of rejection to block your path to self-discovery.

The cost of this plan is some time spent alone, thinking about who you really are and in what you truly believe. This is indeed a job to be approached with fear and trembling. (I often deal with such things while jogging, on the theory that I'm already miserable!) The good news is that while this task is often uncomfortable, it is rarely fatal.

This approach means fewer Great Ideas will be tried. It also means fewer will be abandoned, with the bitter taste of ashes and the sense of failure that accompany lost hopes. Also missing is the wasting of time, energy, and most important in its absence, the weakened bonds of trust which are the offsprings of incongruent behavior.

Can none of these Great Ideas we are forced to abandon ever become a part of your office and life? Certainly! People grow and change, sometimes slowly, deliberately, by their own efforts, other times quickly, almost by accident. (This is more elegantly described as growth by crisis or lysis.) But be warned. Something must cause a very real change in your values to allow these desired, but previously inconsistent ideas, an opportunity for inclusion in your life. Attempted counterfeiting of values will only lead to the failure and frustration we've previously described.

Another way to state this: we can choose to be proactive in our lives, to deliberately subordinate our feelings and desires to our values. This is decidedly not an easy task, but let me caution you: a life lived where short-term gains in feelings are allowed to win the battle over personal commitment and values is a life filled with pain and sadness. Each choice based on a short-term consideration will yield a debt you're allowed to pay in the long term. As tough as a self-aware life is to lead, it's a piece of cake when compared to living a life of self-deceit.

So take heart. As with any worthy goal, achieving your desires will not be easy. In the case of value clarification, be it for your office, or your personal life, this difficulty is certainly real. But the task *can* be accomplished. The rewards, in quality of life and the peace gained from acting consistently with your true values, make the victory well worth the struggle.

CHAPTER 12

THE STOPWATCH:
A DENTIST'S
BEST FRIEND

I bet all of you thought your best friend was your dog. Well, when I'm hunting (which is every chance I get, but never often enough), I agree. However, I'd like to attempt to persuade you that in our offices, the most valuable instrument we can employ may be a stopwatch! That's correct, the office MVP (most valuable possession) is not our beloved high-speed handpiece with the neat little fiber optic light, or even our composite curing light (in that lovely shade of blue), or any of the other gadgets so near and dear to our little dental hearts. None of them, valuable as they are, has so great a potential power to reduce stress, increase income, and generally make our lives in the office both more efficient and pleasant as the humble stopwatch.

I know this is outrageous! You love your high-speed handpiece and all the other marvels of dental technology, as well you should. But let me answer your unspoken question, with a question of my own. What business that manages to remain extant doesn't know exactly how much time each procedure they perform requires? I submit that none do, with the exception of "modern" medicine. The typical medical practice has the singular distinction of being the least timely industry ever to exist. We aren't talking Swiss watch precision or German-train efficiency in the medical offices I've been forced to frequent! This is certainly not the example dentistry chooses to emulate.

Just how much does the timeliness of other industries affect our lives? Do you care if the fast food place of your choice cooks the fries for 10 minutes or an hour? I guess you care only if you eat them. Do you think automotive companies just sort of mess around until a car is manufactured? Does it bother you, just a little, to wait an hour (with your clothes off) to see your friendly physician? Now the telling question: how long does it take you to fabricate a three-surface composite restoration, and *how do you know?*

Allow me to share a parable with you. What follows is a true story from the first days a stopwatch became numbered among my best dental friends and allies.

Years ago I heard a speaker discussing the virtues and advantages of timing every dental procedure. This suggestion was based on his assumption that it would be somehow helpful to precisely know such information. But I already knew. If I didn't have times for procedures clearly recorded, how could my staff properly schedule them? Still, the speaker seemed to believe this timing a worthy enterprise, and I had paid a great deal to travel and hear his presentation, so I invested in a stopwatch.

For most new ideas in my office, I order the materials necessary to implement the new concept, and by the time all the proper equipment has arrived, I've forgotten what I wanted them for. However, in this case we obtained a stopwatch immediately and actually timed a procedure! It so happened that the first treatment to appear on our schedule was an anterior root canal. A simple one-appointment procedure for which I had historically allotted 60 minutes of my time. This had been the time allocated for a single canal endodontic since the day I opened my office. Some time before our first day of seeing patients in my practice, I had *made these times up*. We began our timing after good anesthetic was obtained and stopped the watch when the one-step endodontic fill with gutta percha was completed, but before we began the restoration. The stopwatch showed 13 minutes!

Now I'm not great at math, but I knew that to be under an hour. Could I really do four root canals in the time I had scheduled for one?

Could I make four times the income and still stay on schedule? The 10 years or so since this parable actually took place have answered that query with an emphatic *yes!*

Well, by now my interest in the stopwatch was piqued (as I hope yours has been). We placed 3" x 5" cards in each operatory, with a separate card for each different dental procedure we performed. Each card was marked on the upper edge with the procedure's name. On these cards we recorded a description of the procedure done and the time required to complete it. (For example, on our amalgam card would be an entry MOD—18 minutes.) That was all the information required for our purpose.

We didn't measure the time required to administer local anesthetic, but blocked 10 minutes (the smallest block of time available then in our appointment book) before every procedure requiring the patient be numbed. The time for anesthetic differs greatly from patient to patient, depending on the number of areas to be anesthetized, apprehension level, and cooperation of the patient, among other variables. I never rush in administering anesthetic. Painless injections (or as close to that as is physically possible) are critical to an office's success (much more on painless injections next chapter). It seems this 10-minute average works out well in our office: Some patients require more time, some less, but the needed times seem to balance out in the course of the day. I do want to make it clear that we didn't measure the time required to give anesthetic, but estimated the time required empirically. Such an approach may or may not be adequate for your office needs.

My assistant would start the stopwatch the second we began the actual procedure and stop it the instant it was completed. We didn't measure time to seat the patient, clean rooms, or escort the patient to the front office. We have multiple assistants and rooms, so in our office we have a great deal of flexibility in how these important details are handled. If I operated from one chair or with one chairside assistant, I might wish to record operatory preparation and cleanup times also.

For amalgam and composite restorations, we worked on a basis of surfaces restored per minute. If we performed an MOD, DO, F, and MO in a total of 40 minutes, that is eight surfaces restored, or five minutes per surface. Thus, when we wished to schedule six surfaces of amalgam to be restored we knew we needed 40 minutes—6 surfaces x 5 minutes per surface + 10 minutes for anesthesia. If times didn't figure out to even 10-minute units, *we always rounded numbers up*, because I was scared to death of being rushed. With everything except amalgam and composites we just timed the length of the procedures themselves and averaged those times.

It should have taken a week to gather this information. It took us a couple of months. We often forgot to begin timing, forgot to stop timing, or forgot about timing completely. When we finally did time enough procedures to get what I felt was adequate data, I simply averaged out the times for each procedure, dividing total minutes by number of procedures done. These figures were recorded on a little postcard-sized piece of paper we call our scheduling ruler (a sample is at end of chapter). Thus all the information needed to schedule anything we performed in the office was easily accessible on this one small card.

Today we have multiple doctors working in our office, each with his own scheduling ruler. We schedule from nine computer terminals, so *all* the staff must know exactly how much time is required, not only for each procedure, but for each individual doctor. Without our simple rulers, this could be very difficult to do consistently and correctly, especially when changes or additions to staff personnel are made.

The times required for each procedure vary greatly from doctor to doctor, as they should. The point of timing is not to do any procedure faster, but to schedule work at the ideal pace which allows for performance at the absolute top-quality level of each operator. We aren't recording this information in an attempt to increase our speed chairside. We simply wanted to know how much time is needed for each operator to perform every task to the maximum of his/her ability.

Before I became friends with my little stopwatch buddy, I would look at the schedule for the upcoming day and know that on this day I would have time to spare or that I was really going to be under a lot of time pressure. I'd know this for sure before the day began. I guess this is an example of subconscious awareness, even if we refuse to allow the conscious mind to exactly name the problem. I bet most of you can do the same with your schedule now. Such an awareness just illustrates that you already know when your scheduling is inaccurate. The question is, *How long will you live with this inefficiency before you correct it?*

I'm a hard guy to get along with (as anybody in my office will be happy to tell you). It really bugs me to sit around without a patient. I keep seeing overhead dollars jumping a fence like sheep. But worse than sitting, I *hate* to be behind schedule, even by five minutes. I mean, I really hate it! With my personality, proper scheduling was vital, if for no better reason than to maintain my staff's sanity. (I'll be the first to admit that the state of my staff's sanity is tenuous on a good day. At least their rush to the sanitarium isn't being accelerated due to poor scheduling and its subsequent effect on my moods.)

I've included a copy of part of my personal scheduling ruler for you to peruse. Its virtue lies in its simplicity. The times I use are just that: *my* times. They aren't good or bad, fast or slow. They aren't meant for an example of how much time your procedures should be scheduled for. Your new stopwatch friend will tell you that.

Is it a pain in the rear (pardon the intrusion of complex medical terminology) to time procedures? Yes. Is it worth the trouble? I guess that depends. Would you like to remain on schedule, each and every day? How would your staff and patients feel about that? (Did someone say shocked? Shame on you. I believe an office running according to schedule is as critical to its success as any one factor in a dental practice can possibly be.) Would it save a little of your stomach lining not to have upset patients and staff due to your being "a little behind schedule," to have a normal lunch hour every day, and, barring emergencies, to leave on time every night? Would you like to enjoy the income possible from using your skills at their absolute peak of efficiency? If the answer to any of the previous questions is *yes*, you need a stopwatch.

I don't know if this is directly on the topic, but I want to share with you one other scheduling technique that has greatly improved the quality of my life. Every morning I schedule a 20-minute coffee break! We rarely run behind schedule, but sometimes a patient arrives late, I have to retake an impression, or I have trouble with anesthetic. I love having this time to act as a buffer. If we do get behind schedule, I know we'll be caught up by the end of my break time. Usually I have a cup of coffee and a cookie (I'm perhaps too honest, but it's just one cookie). I take off my shoes and read the paper or the mail. I don't return calls. This is *my break!* Heaven help the staff member whose scheduling causes me to miss this 20 minutes even once. At the end of this respite I brush my teeth and return to my duties, a happier dentist than when I left. I love it!

All the afore-mentioned benefits will occur once you make a commitment to measure your behavior. That's all timing is: a simple measurement of what you're already doing. Think about your feelings looking at the day's schedule. Do you already know intuitively when you have adequate time and when you don't? Now you will have the information needed to get rid of both the slow and the rushed days forever.

I speak with a lot of dentists. I only know of one other doctor that has ever timed all his procedures. Some of the doctors that work with me have chosen not to make the small effort needed to so greatly improve their efficiency. Please let me assure you this will be the most productive time you'll ever spend as a manager in your office. Nothing I can think of grants such a huge benefit that will continue to bear fruit for years at such a small expense in time and money.

I believe that you will find, as I did, greatly reduced stress from being consistently on schedule, a significant increase in income, and a *happier staff and patient group to spend your days with*. There is only one obstacle. You have to do it! Please don't let your own inertia keep you from this simple task.

SAMPLE SCHEDULING RULER

Multiple Amalgams		4 min. per surface
Multiple Composites		6 min. per surface
Anterior/Bicuspid Crown Prep		30 min.
Molar Crown Prep		40 min.
Seat Crown		20 min.
ENDODONTICS	1 Canal	20 min.
	2 Canals	30 min.
	3 Canals	60 min.

This is just a brief sample of my own personal ruler. Remember that we allow 10 minutes for anesthetic for each procedure where it is required. I believe you can see how every procedure you perform can be easily recorded on a single postcard. The system *must* be simple to be used. All procedures done by an assistant or in hygiene are recorded in a similar manner on each of our scheduling rulers, such as Orthodontic Records, 60 minutes; or 4 Sealants, 30 minutes.

Please get that stopwatch today. At your next team meeting share this vision of a more efficient office. Inspire your staff with your vision (lunch on time!). This is a simple team exercise that can change the life of every member of your staff for the better.

CHAPTER 13

THE GREATEST
PRACTICE BUILDER

(That No One Talks About)

Over the years I've been taught or shown so many ways to build my dental practice (and thus avoid the dreaded "busyness monster"), it's a wonder the walls can hold the farrago of patients that's been enticed in. If I become only slightly more behaviorally correct, I'll be in danger of transcendence! And I guess the ideas work—at least I've always been busy.

I've asked patients sincerely and pleasantly to refer their family and friends (we've tried this idea at least). I've conducted exit interviews, published newsletters, got on the patient's level (except for a Vietnamese gentleman who once squatted on the floor—I just don't have the knees). Roses have been sent, flowers given to the favorite patient of the day, special costumes worn on holidays, and zany events held. (Funny Hat Day was a hoot, but the Santa suit got very warm, and trying to work in that large, hot drooping hat—forget it!)

My intent isn't to pooh-pooh these fine methods of practice enhancement (well, maybe just a *little* it is), but to focus on a subject much more critical to practice growth, yet one rarely discussed. It's the art of *gentle, profound, and predictable anesthesia.*

The next time *your* teeth are being treated, ask yourself, "Do I want a rose out of the deal? Or would I rather it didn't hurt?" (If that's a tough question, take your time, but get a response before we go on.)

My admittedly informal survey (I asked my staff) was strongly biased toward *don't hurt!* (However, I have discovered that one of my staff has been way too long between roses!) Ask around and see if most people don't tell you the same thing.

But don't all doctors give "gentle, profound, and predictable anesthesia?" No, at least not according to some of the patients I see. One sweet lady in her 70s told me, "That's the first shot I've gotten in my life that didn't hurt." (Seventy years is a long time to wait—for anything.) Do you think there is a chance she mentioned this event to anyone else? Is it *possible* the people she mentioned it to didn't like injections that hurt either? If you have $5, you can get a rose, but a shot that doesn't hurt can be hard to come by.

I believe most doctors really think, "My shots don't hurt" (not much at least), but start to *observe* your patients. Do they tense up, close their eyes, or occasionally kick their feet and scream? All these behaviors could be subtle clues that things aren't as comfortable as you'd hoped. Possibly I'm unique, but I can feel the tension in a patient, and *it doesn't feel good.* Their pulse becomes my pulse and their blood pressure, mine. And you, doctor, get to do this 10–20 times a day. The patient at least only has to put up with it once.

This brings me to a second major point about anesthesia: "gentle, profound, and predictable anesthesia" can save or at least prolong a life: yours. Nothing in dentistry is as stressful to me as treating a patient who can "feel it," or even a patient who suspects they may be about to "feel it."

I once traveled 200 miles to watch a noted specialist at work (both to learn from this great man and to avoid my own patients for a day). During the course of their day, they opened and drained an abscess for an emergency patient. The procedure didn't take long, but she "felt it." When the abscess was opened and the screaming and kicking had stopped, I found myself out in the hall with sweat on my lip and a really bad headache. Thank God I was only watching.

To me, the most amazing part of this whole scenario was the behavior of patients in the reception room: they were still there! Such unhappy occurrences are not good for dentistry or for the dentist, staff, and patient involved.

So I hope you'll grant me these two points:

1. Treating patients without good anesthesia or hurting them during the injection is stressful for everybody in the room. It's something we'd like to avoid, if for no other reason than to save wear and tear on our own gastric lining.

2. The ability to provide gentle, profound, predictable anesthesia may be the biggest practice builder there is (or lack of this skill may have the biggest negative impact on a practice possible). My 20-plus years of clinical experience have allowed me to become acquainted with a lot of people whose former dentist hurt them. As most of us don't want to be the next former dentist, let's explore exactly how to avoid this fate.

Let me begin with this disclaimer: I'm no expert on local anesthetic. On the other hand, I do possess a secret weapon. I have the good fortune to be terrified of needles (the sharp, pointy end, at least). This has given me an empathy that borders on the supernatural and explains my own selfish reasons for trying so hard not to cause any discomfort when injections are given.

That said, I believe we have two separate subjects to address:

1. Gentle anesthesia, and

2. Profound and predictable anesthesia.

GENTLE

I've often wondered, do my patients love me, or is it my nitrous oxide? I suppose if nitrous oxide sedation were outlawed, I'd still practice dentistry, but I try not to think about things like that. I certainly can't explain to you all of the techniques involved in the use of nitrous oxide in this format, but I think nitrous is a critical ingredient for painless injections.

We don't use nitrous on every patient. Some just don't need it, or they dislike the sensation. A few won't tolerate their noses being covered. Also, the percentage of nitrous we give during injections can vary from

12% to 50%, depending on the patient. A feel for this right amount takes time and experience. However, most local anesthetic (even the mandibular block) can be given with no discomfort, thanks to the help of the proper dosage of "laughing gas" and the other technique tips that follow.

This next point seems to be somewhat controversial, but I treat a ton of kids, and despite the marvels of fluoride and sealants, they still get a cavity or two. *It has been years since I've needed to use local anesthetic on a primary tooth,* unless a vital pulpotomy or extraction was indicated. Instead of using local while treating children, I use 5 liters of oxygen and 4 liters of nitrous for anesthesia. The only time a patient will experience discomfort is if they are "sneaking" breaths out of their mouth (and some little kids can be very subtle at this behavior).

If a child is mouth breathing, you must stop a minute (literally about 60 seconds) and be sure they are breathing through the "elephant nose" (our cute name for the nitrous nosepiece).

This mouth breathing is usually only a problem with some three- or four-year-olds, and then only for the first time they are treated. Once they get used to the nosepiece and the pleasant, relaxing sensation, there's no problem getting them to breathe correctly.

The use of stereo headphones also helps a lot. Having your nose covered by a nosepiece can be sort of scary when you're three years old. We use bubble gum–flavored nosepieces, but my colleague on tape, Dr. Winnie the Pooh, is my best helper to get kids to forget the nosepiece and relax. I'm sure Dr. Pooh isolates the child from some unpleasant auditory stimulation as well. While music or any other tape can help, my advice is to never underestimate the power of Pooh!

I've had doctors tell me for 15 years, "You can't use just nitrous to work on primary teeth." I do it every day and so do the doctors that work with me. If giving anesthetic to three-year-olds is your idea of a good time, be my guest. If not, you really should give this a try. Next time you pass through Keokuk, Iowa (it's pretty much on line with Paris), stop in, and some kid and I will give you a demonstration.

My next best "gentle" helper is a good topical anesthetic, place on dried tissue for a few seconds. I've had doctors tell me topicals just don't reduce discomfort. It's really very easy to find out. Just give yourself a little local (you big chicken), and use topical on one side and not on the other. There's no reason you should take my word for it, and this experiment should eliminate all doubt as to topicals' effectiveness. We use Sultan Topex, but I think most topicals work well. I select them more on the basis of smell and taste, as they all seem to provide good topical anesthesia.

I always wiggle the tissue vigorously while placing the needle and injecting, especially during mandibular blocks. As I understand it, this concept is part of the "gate" theory of pain. If the nerves are carrying a movement or pressure message to the brain, they can't carry the "ouch" message.

The last point about *gentle* is the most critical: *go slowly*. After a while you can gauge the proper injection speed by the patient's reactions. If you go too quickly, you'll feel the patient tense. I've watched lots of dentists give anesthetic, and they're always a lot faster at injecting than I am. After the injection, they wait for the anesthetic to take effect (and for the patient's back to straighten—the "Don't-treat-them-until-their-butt-is-back-in-the-chair" method, I guess).

It's much better to inject very slowly and carry on a conversation as you're injecting to help distract the patient. (If you know that his wife is having an affair, mentioning it during the injection would be an almost perfect distraction.) It's a little hard at first to find something to talk about at a tension-filled time like this, but with experience and effort, this conversational distraction can become second nature too. Focusing the patient's mind on anything other than the tip of the needle helps.

PROFOUND AND PREDICTABLE

Here I'm really not an expert, but I thought I'd tell you a few little things I do that may help.

1. Occasionally upper molars, especially second and third molars, won't get numb, even for routine operative, without palatal anesthesia. When a couple of buccal infiltrations haven't been effective, palatal anesthetic usually numbs the tooth almost instantly. When giving a palatal, I place a topical, push hard over the foramen area with my fingertip for a few seconds, give the anesthetic, and then tell the patient I'm sorry, because it almost always hurts, and I really am sorry. I tell the patient I'd rather

hurt them this one time instead of having discomfort every time I touch the tooth. (Maybe somebody's got a better answer for palatal anesthetic and will write me. I've tried the anesthetic "guns" for this procedure, and it seems to feel somewhat more comfortable, but it scares patients with a popping noise.)

2. To achieve anesthesia painlessly on the maxillary central incisors, I inject over the canine, wait a minute and then infiltrate over the central I'm going to treat. If you go slowly, this doesn't hurt, and the patient is usually amazed, as past injections in this sensitive area were so painful (from that former guy).

3. Mandibular blocks can be the real posers. Here are the techniques I use in the sequence in which they are employed.

    a. Gow-Gates block. I've used it routinely for years. It's safer and more comfortable, in my opinion. It's also simple to learn.

    b. Routine mandibular block. If the patient is jumpy I may give both the Gow-Gates and conventional block before I even begin a procedure.

    c. Buccal and mental infiltration. If I were doing multiple crowns or molar endo on a new patient or a nervous one, I may use all three of these techniques to begin with. I'm not really recommending that. I know it's a lot of anesthesia and medically may not be the wisest, but I really like my patients to be free of all discomfort. (No one ever says, "I think I was too numb." If they're not numb enough, they may mention it.)

    d. Lingual infiltration. This I rarely need, usually just for endo or removal of a lower molar. The lingual bone is much thinner on the mandible than the buccal plate of bone, so infiltration on the lingual is more effective.

    e. Ligajet. When all these aren't enough on a tooth scheduled for removal or endo, I use the ligajet. I choose not to use this on teeth that are to remain vital, and I don't use it until the soft tissue is already numb. In my clumsy hands, the ligajet seems to be more painful than the conventional syringe. It does, however, almost always give instant anesthetic, even on the toughest of teeth, the sore lower molar. However, the ligajet is least effective on mandibular molars, especially ones with very long roots.

So there you have it, a few diamonds from the creek bed of experience. I believe that taking the time to be really concerned about patient comfort—and gentle, profound local anesthetic is certainly only one way among many you can show your concern—is really the greatest practice builder, one we should all think and talk about.

For some of you, an increase in skill or technique may be required, but for most experienced doctors, I believe it is only a matter of carefully considering the benefits to them, their practice, and patients. For many patients the single biggest concern of any dental appointment, more than fee, convenience, or pleasantness of the staff, is, "Will it hurt?" It's very possible for you to look them in the eye and say, "No, it will not." Sure, it will take a little more time and effort on your part to keep this promise, but if you or a loved one were the patient, wouldn't it be worth it?

CHAPTER 14

EXPANDED HYGIENE: A WINNING CONCEPT FOR EVERYONE

What would you say if I told you that in just a few months we could end the national hygienist shortage? If I informed you that your production and profitability could increase while your hygienist's income grew and her stress dropped, would you be interested? What if, by making this change, both the amount of service and the professionalism of the care to your patients were improved? Would you be intrigued enough to wish to hear more?

The answer to all the above questions is *expanded hygiene*. Not a new concept, but one mostly overlooked in dentistry today. Here's how the system works: To achieve all the benefits mentioned above, your hygienist must have available for her use at all times two fully equipped hygiene rooms and her own assistant.

As your hygienist is caring for her first patient in Room 1, her assistant is seating another patient in Room 2, which is already cleaned and set up in advance. The assistant now helps the patient review or fill out a medical history, takes blood pressures, or exposes any needed

X-rays. She can make sure the patient is comfortable, and answer any questions they may have.

The hygienist completes the needed care on the patient in the first room and enters Room 2. With no delay she can begin treatment of the patient awaiting her there.

The assistant moves back to Room 1 where she polishes and flosses the first patient (law allowing). She reviews oral hygiene or the use of any oral hygiene aids selected by the hygienist. She has plenty of time to interact with the patient and answer questions or explain suggested treatment. She schedules the next appointment (if you do this in hygiene) and escorts the patient to the front desk. She returns, cleans the operatory to the best OSHA-approved standards, and seats the next patient. This cycle is repeated throughout the day.

Why go to all this bother? Two rooms and an assistant, just for hygiene? Well, let's take a look at some numbers. (Please bear in mind, the figures used here are, as we writers say, "made up." Get out a pencil and paper and substitute your own fees and salaries for these fabricated ones to see how effectively this premise will work in your office.)

Say your current excellent hygienist treats eight patients a day and earns a salary of $18 per hour, or $144 for an eight-hour day. Let's also assume that each patient receives a simple prophy for $24, a fluoride treatment for $15, and a recall exam at $15. That's a total of $54 per patient times eight patients per day or $432 of total hygiene production each day. Take away the salary of $144 and you have $288 left over to pay the rent.

To make this example simple, we'll leave out X-rays, sealants, perio procedures, as well as failed and canceled appointments and people who don't pay their bills. (In our office, panos, treatment of periodontal disease, and placement of sealants are probably the most financially rewarding procedures performed in the hygiene department. We exclude them to simplify the example, but elimination of these larger production procedures makes our final figures very conservative.)

Our expanded hygienist in this example still gets a $144 daily salary. She now has an assistant who gets as an entry level wage of $6 an hour, or $48 per day. Total salary for the two staff is now $192 per day. Together they see 12 patients a day (The two working together can easily treat this number of extra patients). Which group gets the most attention? The eight patients treated in eight hours of care time or the 12 patients cared for in 16 hours of staff time?

At our arbitrary fee of $54 per patient, that's $648 production. (Our office hygiene production is stable around $98 per hour, or $784 daily, so $648 is a conservative estimate.) Remove the $192 salary from this total, and you have $456 remaining vs. the $288 of the unassisted hygiene system. That is a $168 per day difference after all salaries are paid. If your hygienist works 200 days per year, that means an additional $36,000/year remains.

Take a minute to study your office overhead without salaries. This percentage (total overhead percentage minus salary overhead percentage) times the extra dollars produced gives you the additional *net income* per day you earn as the manager who set up this system. But, more than this, if hygiene is seeing 50% more patients, what does that do to the doctor's production as more needed care is diagnosed?

(To save you curious people a little time, if you take our office's actual daily hygiene production of $784 and remove $192 in salaries, you have $592 remaining. Reduce this figure by the $288 per day an unassisted hygienist can produce, and you have $304 per day, or $60,000 per year of additional income based on a 200-day working year.

Our overhead minus all salaries is 35%, so my net income is increased by 65% of this $60,000, or roughly $39,500. You all know how near and dear old *net* is to this boy's heart. All this assumes you have the patient load to fill the hygiene book at this new level of treatment efficiency.)

We've used this system for seven years. Initially, our hygienist was frightened of "becoming a scaling machine" and suffering burnout. It just isn't so. Fatigue comes mostly from all the little jobs like taking, developing, and mounting X-rays, or the drudgery of repeating over and over things like oral-hygiene instructions and room cleanup and setup.

Another big benefit is that the hygienist, her assistant, and the front-office person who schedules most of the hygiene patients become part of a team with common goals. They keep their own monitors of the hygiene department and have their own staff meetings (as we've discussed). I suspect "team member" is a pleasant change from the lonely job description of "the hygienist."

The hygiene assistant must be selected carefully. A real "people person" is needed (a very outgoing individual with outstanding communication skills). She must be committed to the patients' health and well-being and show that she really cares about their dental health and about them as people. The treatment part of her job is not nearly as complex and involved as what must be learned by the doctor's chairside, so in hiring for this position, I consider a sparkling, outgoing personality to be by far the most important requirement.

Procedurally, our hygiene assistant will take any needed X-rays and study models; do the polishing, flossing and fluoride treatments; give all oral hygiene instructions, review the medical histories, and perform all sterilization of instruments, room cleanup, and setup. In our office she also makes all custom trays and takes 90% of our orthodontic records.

Our hygiene assistant has also proven to be a valuable asset filling in as the doctor's chairside assistant when we need her. Developing skills at chairside work helps her to better understand restorative dentistry and allows her to answer questions concerning needed care with authority (as well as bailing us out if we need extra help).

It didn't take us too long, working in this expanded fashion, to realize the huge difference in production this was making in our practice. We looked for a system of compensation that would both motivate the hygiene department to perform at an even higher level of efficiency and reward them equitably when they did so.

To establish a system of remuneration for our hygiene people that would reward them based on how much actual treatment they performed (as opposed to hours of work they showed up for), we took the total hygiene production of the hygienist and her assistant for the previous 12 months and divided it into each person's total salary for that same period. (This total salary includes all paid benefits they had been compensated for such as sick leave, vacation, etc.; these perquisites are now included in our percentage figure and don't need to be dealt with individually.)

Say for example, the hygiene department produced $100,000 in the last 12 months, and during that time our hygienist compensation including all benefits was $22,000. We now have a percentage of 22 to base future compensation on. Similar calculations were done for the assistant. (They are a team, and the last thing you'd desire is one team member who gets extra money for doing additional work, while the other team member is paid the same, whether working harder or not.) Their compensation is now this calculated percentage of their future production. The more they produce, the more money they make (hey, just like me!). When no patient is being treated, they aren't being paid (like me again), and *they have a problem*. (Doesn't it bug you to see your hygienist having a cup of coffee and being paid her full salary when a patient wasn't there to treat? Now, you may be paying for the cup of coffee, but her time is her own. It sure makes me feel better!)

I don't wish to give you actual percentages or dollar figures from our office. The final dollar figures that will emerge in your practice will be determined by your patient load, management ability within your team, and the motivation and skill of your staff. Our hygiene staff raised their salaries 20% immediately when this system was introduced by working harder. You could argue that they should have worked that hard before they were on a commission. It seems to me nothing more than human nature to work harder if you know you will receive extra compensation commensurate to your labors. It also seems to me the job of a leader to create such a self-motivational system, because you profit at least as much as your staff does by the increases in their production.

I've heard objections to paying hygienists based on commission— that they might hurry through just to increase their income, not be as gentle, or not do as thorough a job. This theory seems to suggest that hygienists are less moral than dentists who could do the same thing during their patient care, or that hygienists are less far-sighted because they don't realize patients are lost to the office by such practices, and in the long run lost patients hurt everyone. But even if this concern were valid, do you think you wouldn't notice tartar left on teeth, or be aware of patients hurt and leaving? In 20-plus years of private practice and the five hygienists I've worked with, the quality of their care has yet to be a problem.

Expanded hygiene benefits the patients because they're in our office a full hour for a cleaning with trained staff attending them continually. Both the hygienists and especially the assistant have plenty of time to educate, reinforce suggestions, and make friends—maybe even to recommend possible treatment needed and stress the value of regular professional cleanings.

There are some disadvantages. You have to have two fully equipped treatment rooms. Our two hygiene rooms have nitrous oxide, stereo headphones, X-rays and every convenience available in any other operatory in our office.

I strongly suggest that you become skilled at periodontal care (there are a lot of good nonsurgical perio courses around for general dentists), with full-mouth surveys, full-mouth charting of pockets and excellent documentation becoming the norm on every periodontal patient seen in your office. With the legal climate as it is today, this would seem good advice to any office, but as your hygiene people seek ways to grow in their ability to offer treatment, it may become even more imperative in your office.

However, charting is much easier and faster with an assistant to record pocket depths, and a chairside with a suction makes heavily bleeding periodontal procedures much easier to perform. I believe it is *essential* that whoever does sealants in your office have a chairside available while placing them. Sealants don't perform well if placed in Lake Saliva, especially if done at high tide.

These problems are more than made up for by all the advantages we've discussed. The patients win because more time and care are devoted to them at *the same fee*, so value given to your patients is increased. They never feel they are being rushed. The concern of the staff for them as people is evident.

The hygienist wins because she is free to use her unique professional skills and not be tied up in the drudgery and tedium of jobs that we dentists have delegated for years. (When was the last time you scrubbed instruments? Do you miss all that fun?) She is part of a professional team and no longer feels isolated from the rest of the staff. I personally believe this isolation is why so many hygienists leave the profession after just a few years. Due to all the features we have mentioned, she has reduced stress and, if she chooses to work harder, a significantly increased income.

The doctor wins because hygiene is more productive, more professional, and more profitable. Seeing extra patients means more restorative care will be diagnosed. Both the increased hygiene production and the additional treatment recommended lead to an increase in revenue for the practice. For all these reasons, dentistry wins! Isn't that a pleasant thought?

One concern may remain. As exciting as all this sounds (and if it doesn't sound exciting, you'd better read it again), you may be uncertain whether your practice has the patient load to support such an accelerated treatment system.

This is a valid concern, especially if you are already having difficulty keeping your hygiene department busy. You don't want to place them on a commission system of compensation, only to realize they're losing money due to decreasing patient demand. This is not the formula for a happy dental team!

Also, you need to be very sure a hygiene *team* exists (including the hygienist, her assistant, and the person scheduling most hygiene appointments) before this system is implemented. It is essential that everyone on the team be committed to a common goal if the plan is to have any opportunity for success. Be sure that every member of this group completely understands and accepts the roles expanded hygiene will mean to them before attempting to implement the system.

Our office solved any possible busyness problem by *plugging our patient leaks.* I guess all practices have "cracks" that patients fall through. Through these flaws in your recall apparatus, your most valuable single commodity, the patients who have already chosen you to perform their dental care slowly trickle away.

Our first step in the "caulking process" was to have hygiene schedule their own recalls, because the people working in hygiene are more committed than anyone else in the office to having patients return for regular preventive care. This higher level of commitment should be due to their professional belief in the need for the treatment they provide, as well as a natural desire to be well-compensated personally in our new financial arrangement. Our nine-terminal computer system makes it simple for recare to be scheduled by our hygiene assistant while the patients are still in the operatory. I'm sure an appointment book will work as well. Whatever method of scheduling you use, both the doctor and the hygiene department must have their work calendar (a listing of what days they will be seeing patients in the office) completed for at least 12 months in advance, so this prebooking can be accomplished.

I've tried a lot of recall systems over the years. Scheduling patients while they are in your office receiving their current care is by far the most effective. The patients can choose the day of the week and the time of day best for their personal schedules. We call patients three days before the scheduled prebooked appointment to confirm that this time will still be acceptable to them. If someone needs to make a change from the prebooked appointment they selected at the time of their last treatment, we have ample time to fill our schedule.

The next step in our quest to reconnect with these vital patients (whose loss so attenuated our office vitality) was to implement what we call our *chart audit system*. We have one staff person who spends about eight hours a week going through records and identifying patients who are past due for dental care. These patients are called personally, and our concern for their dental health is expressed. The first statement made to such a prodigal patient is always, "Hi, Sue. This is Carol from Dr. Wilde's office. Dr. Wilde has asked me to call. He's concerned about you. Did you know it has been _____ since your last visit to our office?"

There is a great deal of *power* in the message that the doctor has asked that you be called, that he or she is concerned. Usually patients will schedule an appointment and are surprised at how long it has been since their last care. Occasionally they inform us they know they are overdue, but this is a bad time for them. They ask if we could call them back in the future. A note is made, and placed in a special tickler file. At the time they have requested (usually a month or two), we call and see if they are now ready to resume care.

We sometimes find a patient has chosen to leave our practice. If they have decided to seek care elsewhere, we thank them for allowing us to be of service. We wish them well, offer to transfer copies of their records and X-rays to the office of their choice free of charge, and assure them we'd love to see them again if we can ever be of service.

The records of patients choosing to go elsewhere for dental care are placed on my desk, with a brief note detailing the reason for their departure. I send them a letter expressing our thanks for the trust in us they have shown by choosing our office to help with their oral health care and offering them best wishes and our continued support.

This office policy creates as much of a positive event out of a negative incident (i.e., patients leaving) as possible. I always feel a little hurt when a patient leaves our care, but mastery is performing at your best in *difficult times*. How your team handles patient rejection is a good barometer of your professionalism and your true concern for the well-being of your patients.

I also like to be aware of the reasons people leave, painful as this may be, in the hope that I can identify any office policies that may be the cause of patient desertion. Spotting such a trend may allow us to make adjustments in a policy resulting in our office being able to retain more patients.

I believe most doctors prefer not to hear about patients who chose to go elsewhere for care. If they do receive this unpleasant information, there is a tendency to be defensive and search for reasons why the patient's leaving wasn't "our fault." This common behavior ignores a vital source of feedback to help your office improve. A skilled staff person can identify what made the patient decide to transfer from your office. It may be something unavoidable, but sometimes a pattern can be detected that could potentially be damaging to the well-being of the office. The sooner it can be corrected, the better for all.

Sometimes a misunderstanding between a team member and a particular patient has caused the problem, and if this can be rectified by a skilled staff member, the patient and his/her good will can be retained. I understand the reluctance to study patients who have chosen to leave your care. It's very natural to feel somewhat defensive. But remember, successful people choose to do what less successful people refuse to do. You can learn a great deal from the patients who leave you, if you can approach the subject in an open and positive manner.

In addition to making phone calls to reestablish relationships with patients out of touch with our office, our chart auditor also sends a form offering a free exam to people who have been at least two years out of contact with our office. X-rays are not included in the no-charge offer. It amazes me how many people will accept the examination appointment, seemingly enticed by the fact there will be no charge for this service and then schedule for hundreds of dollars of needed care, after we have completed a careful codiagnosis. It's just human nature to like a bargain I guess.

The person doing the chart auditing can be any member of the staff who has outstanding communication and people skills. A knowledge of dentistry and of our office and its policies allows her to answer patient questions intelligently. It doesn't matter if our chart auditor works in our front office or chairside, as long as she possesses these needed skills. We once hired someone from outside our office to do chart audit only. Despite a history of years in the dental field, her lack of knowledge about us made our office look like all the other "phone solicitation" people who disturb my evenings. It wasn't her fault, but it just didn't work. The chart audit person is an ambassador of your office, and thus an extension of your purpose. She too must reflect the values your office stands for.

The staff person you select for this critical job should be given the time she needs to do this job fully and professionally and not try to squeeze chart audit duties in among her other jobs. *We usually have about 50 patients a month scheduled by our auditing,* and they usually need more care than the patients who keep regular recall appointments. Chart audit is a vital and financially rewarding segment of our office procedure, not a "fill-time" job to be done when a staff member has nothing else that needs to be accomplished.

If you are wondering how long it takes to complete chart auditing, the answer in our office is *forever.* By the time a staff person has gone completely through our 5,000 records, it's time to go back and start once again. Remember, these are patients who have already selected you to care for their oral health needs. It is much easier to reactivate them to your practice than it is to attract new patients. Most of the time they're aware they are overdue for care and just need a little nudge to redirect them.

If you want an idea of how much added hygiene potential exists in your office, have a staff member pull 100 charts at random and see how many of these patients are behind their scheduled recall dates. I have a feeling it will be a real learning experience for you. Once you have obtained this percentage, estimate how many total patients of record you have to get an idea of how many patients are out of commitment with your office.

Let's assume that of the 100 charts you selected, you identify 24 patients who are currently out of commitment with your office (sadly, I think this percentage would be fairly typical). You estimate there are 2,000 total patient records in your files, and 24% of 2,000 means you have 480 patients delinquent for their needed care. If you see 12 hygiene patients a day, that's 40 working days of full hygiene production.

As you begin to contact these folks, you'll soon get an idea of what percentage will actually choose to make appointments at this time and thus can plan what future hygiene load you must prepare for. This should give you enough information to decide if expanded hygiene is feasible in your office.

Here is a copy of the form letter that we send to all patients who have notified us that they will be leaving our practice. Many times these same patients return to us for care at a later date. Often the new office (which usually has lower fees than we do) just doesn't give them the quality of care they have become used to in our environment. I'd like to think this letter makes it easier for them to return, and even if they never do come back to us for care, the last contact they have with our team is a reaffirmation of our caring about them and our commitment to their oral health. We really do care, and we really are committed. The letter just reminds them of these facts.

Dear_____

We're sorry to hear of your request to transfer to another dental office. As always, our main concern is for your dental health. Please continue to make every effort to obtain optimal oral health care. We will be happy to transfer any X-rays or records that will be helpful to you, and if at any time in the future we can be of service to you in any way, please let us know.

Thanks for allowing us to serve your dental needs, and best of luck.

Sincerely,

John A. Wilde, D.D.S., P.C. and Staff

What follows is a copy of the form letter we send to people who have been out of contact with our office for at least two years, as part of the chart audit efforts we discussed earlier in this chapter. You will recall that the examination is free, but not any needed X-rays. I am continually surprised by how many patients accept this offer. Of course, after two or more years with no care, they often need a lot of dental treatment, so even if our response to these letters were as low as 10%, I'd be very pleased to see these folks. After two years they really need our help!

Date
Name and address of patient
Dear_____

After reviewing our records, we find it has been _____ years since your last professional cleaning and oral health examination in our office. Regular check-ups, even when everything seems OK, are a proven way to maintain your teeth for life. Oral cancer, periodontal (gum) diseases, TMJ problems, and new decay are just a few of the disorders that we frequently diagnose during routine well-patient checkups. Because we are concerned about your dental health, we would like to offer you a free exam upon returning this letter within 10 days. Please complete the form below and return it to our office in the enclosed envelope.

☐ I am interested in the free exam. Please call me to set up an appointment. My phone number is _____ and the best time to reach me is _____.

☐ I am not interested. Please remove my name from your active list.

☐ I am going to another dentist. Please forward my records to:_____.

We are looking forward to hearing from you. Thank you, and if you have any questions, please call.

Sincerely,

John A. Wilde D.D.S., P.C. and Staff

We enclose a self-addressed and stamped envelope. People who haven't been to a dentist in over two years have many barriers keeping them away. We want to make things as easy as possible for them to say, "Yes." Of course, if they call after ten days, we are still happy to schedule them. If they ask if other members of their family can have a free exam, we say, "Of course, we'd be honored to see them." We wish to reestablish contact with anyone who needs our care. Once we do a careful exam and codiagnosis, with them holding a mirror, almost everyone returns for all needed treatment.

It's very hard to ignore dental problems once you have observed them in your own mouth. I look forward to the intraoral video cameras as a great adjunct to our care. Personally, I'm patient enough to wait until the quality and price of these worthy devices stabilize. As with computers in the past, these video aids seem to be getting better and cheaper, while some companies that produce them are falling out of the business. I admire people who like to be on the cutting edge of technology, but I've been cut there a time or two myself (I guess today such a laceration could easily be repaired by a laser). A hand-held mirror has worked well for us for years, but there is no question that the video apparatus is the wave of the future. I just plan to delay my purchase until I'm certain the wave I choose to ride won't be crashing into the beach.

Please share this information with your team. The plans contained within this chapter will increase your *net*, enhance your team's compensation, and allow you to provide more and better care for your patients.

Will you choose to pass up a plan with all these benefits? Get your team involved right away.

CHAPTER 15

PROS AND CONS
OF A
SMALL GROUP
PRACTICE

After 11 years of solo practice, I made a decision to select an associate to join our dental team. That decision was made in 1985. Now three of us practice in what for so many years was just my office. The years that have followed my decision to add other providers to our team have contained many delights, but also more than a few horrors. I personally am totally committed to a group concept and would never consider solo practice again. Yet daily I'm aware of all the extra problems a group practice entails, and I often reflect back with "my" staff on the good old days—when it was just us.

I'd like to share with you in as even-handed a manner as possible the advantages and disadvantages of a small group practice. I think, next to marriage, the choice to enter group practice is the biggest decision most professionals make. Let's take a serious look on both sides of the group practice fence.

The critical first step for any doctor is to *clarify why he/she would consider a group*. For me, the pressure of solo practice became just too great. In 1985 our office was collecting $40,000 per month, had 5,000 active patients (by actual record count), and often saw 10 or more emergency patients a day. I had maximized my own productive capabilities with five fully equipped operatories and an excellent, experienced staff of seven, but I still couldn't keep up with the patient demand. The choices were:

1. Get some help, or

2. Turn patients away.

I returned from a week of March skiing in Colorado to be greeted with a list hanging on my office wall. The fateful list contained the names of 45 people who had emergency dental problems. We already had a full schedule for the week. The emergency patients were in pain and already were displeased at having been forced to wait a week for me to return. In the course of the week, we saw about an additional 40 emergency patients who contacted us during the week itself. The skiing had been lovely, but the trip long and fatiguing. I returned tired before my marathon of dental care even began. Somewhere in the course of that week I experienced a moment of epiphany: *I need some help!*

For a young professional just starting in the business of dentistry, reasons to consider joining a group practice may include:

1. A lack of funds to begin your own practice,

2. A desire to have an experienced dentist around to help in the development of your clinical and business skills, or

3. A personal lack of interest in the business aspects of dentistry.

Established doctors may investigate the possibilities of adding an associate because:

1. They desire help in treating an excessive patient load,

2. They would value the sharing of overhead expenses to reduce those pressures, or

3. They would like to build a relationship with someone who one day will wish to buy all or a part of their practice and thus free some equity capital for the owner.

These and many more excellent reasons exist to consider a group practice.

PROS

Since I have chosen to work in a group practice setting, I'll begin with the pros, but I want to caution you that the cons are also compelling. Doctors considering a group must evaluate all the factors we'll discuss, plus many more personal concerns I've not included in our discussion. They must assign a level of personal importance or weight to each factor based on their experiences in an effort to make the best decision for their unique situation.

Let's consider the advantages to group practice:

MORE NEW PATIENTS

With multiple providers we were forced by limited space (five operatories and 2,000 square feet) to stagger our hours of patient care and to offer evening and Saturday appointment times.

The positive side of this change in our working hours was the added patient convenience created. *This single change in our office hours led to a 50% increase in new-patient flow almost immediately after a second doctor joined our practice.* In our community, families with both spouses working and people reluctant to take kids out of school found this added availability very attractive. The presence of another doctor and added staff in the community also led to a greater new patient flow.

Over the years as our office size has varied from two to three doctors, by some alchemy I can't precisely describe, the flow of new patients has changed in relation to the number of doctors employed at any given moment in our office. While I can't exactly explain it, all of us are grateful for this occurrence.

LOWER FIXED OVERHEAD

We needed to make almost no changes to our office physical plant when we added an associate. The cost of our heating, cooling, phones, business insurance (not malpractice, of course), and rent stayed pretty much the same. In 1986 our office overhead percentage dropped from 65% (as a solo practitioner with a staff of seven), to 58% with two doctors and nine staff members working in our office. Our average office production went from $40,000 to $60,000 per month.

So many little changes occurred in the transition to a multidoctor practice that it's difficult to establish a figure as our fixed-overhead savings, but I think it's fair to say rent, utilities, and some insurances are cut in half (or into thirds, in our current three-doctor situation), and many other expenses are reduced to a lesser extent.

For example, in 1986, as I mentioned, we went from seven staff members to nine after the addition of our first associate, while our collected dollars went from $40,000 to $60,000 monthly. Working alone, we had produced $5,700 per staff member per month. With an associate's production added, we went to $6,600 per staff member per month. The bottom line, and to me the biggest factor of the group concept, is *more net dollars are left to share among all the doctors involved in the practice.*

I can't overstress this vital point. The total dollars brought into the office increases, while the percentage of overhead drops. This gives a double boost to our net increase: as both increased production and collection, as well as reduced percentage of overhead lead to an increase in my old friend *net profit.*

To use the figures quoted above from our first year with an associate as an example, we went from $40,000 collection per month average and 65% overhead (and thus a $14,000 per month net) to $60,000 per month collections at 58% overhead (and a $25,200 per month net).

Granted, this profit is now split between two doctors.

How much you pay your associate will depend on the geographic area you reside in, your own philosophy, and many other variables, but let's examine these numbers in two other ways. Say your associate produces $20,000 per month (as ours did) and you pay him 30% of the collected total (this was the original contract figure for our first associate). Thus his salary for that month is $6,000 (30% of $20,000). The practice net was $25,200, and less the $6,000 associate earnings, your net is $19,200. *The owner's net has increased $5,200 dollars per month, or $62,400 per year, and your production and time spent chairside have stayed the same.*

Have you "stolen" the money that your poor associate earned by the sweat of his/her—shall we say, brow? Let's examine the numbers again. You have reduced overhead (as good managers should) by 7%. Seven percent of $60,000 is $4,300. So all but $900 of your increased profits comes from your managerial expertise by reducing your costs of doing business.

But even if the entire added profit came from the associate's efforts, I still feel the money was well-earned by the senior dentist. He/she has provided the patient load, the trained staff, as well as the philosophy and vision of success. It is he/she who has made the effort to search and hire the proper person for his office. All these accomplishments makes the owner deserving of a reward.

One last point: this additional profit continues month after month, unless the associate improves his/her skills. Then it increases.

CASH FLOW

Adding new equipment and services becomes much less of a financial burden due to the accelerated production capabilities of a multiprovider office. Adding a panorex or computer system, as well as continuing education expenses, now is more affordable due to the increased cash flow. As the new additions in equipment or services available are now used for more hours and benefit more patients, they also increase profitability to a greater extent than possible in a solo office. In a solo practice, some of these needed additions are difficult to justify financially. It is virtually impossible for a solo practice to keep pace with a group when it comes to updated facilities or marketing efforts. The group is simply making a double or triple return over the solo practitioner on every practice-enhancing investment they make.

MINISPECIALIZATION

In our community of 13,000, the only specialty support is that of a full-time orthodontist and an oral surgeon in town one day per week. I used to do a lot of procedures of a specialty nature to accommodate people (most specialists in our area don't have expanded hours, so a trip to their office could mean a lost day of work as well as travel expenses for our patient). Often these procedures were stressful to me, and I felt they would have been performed at a higher level of quality, with much less attendant effort, by a specialist.

Whether by luck or design, in our current group of three, we have at least one doctor with unusual skills and/or interests in each specialty area of dental practice. (The other doctors have skills; I have interest.) This allows each of us to spend more time performing in the subspecialties of dentistry we enjoy the most. We are allowed to concentrate our energies and talents in those areas we prefer, and thus we are able to provide the patients with a better service based on our expanded experience and studies. Our increased levels of knowledge and skills in our particular areas of expertise make us work more quickly and efficiently. This increase in quality of care justifies an increase in our fee for that service. Of course, both increased efficiency and a higher fee add to our *net*.

As an example, I no longer remove teeth, a job I did reluctantly for years but never enjoyed. This saves patients from my less-than-complete mastery of the art of exodontia. It keeps me from having to do procedures I dislike almost to the point of phobia. It also means another member of our group who, for reasons mysterious to me, enjoys removing teeth, gets to provide more of this service to our patients. Of course, as his skills are greater in this area than mine, the treatment is completed much more quickly. We make more money, and few patients complain that they wish we had pulled their teeth more slowly.

Much of the treatment I referred out in the past now stays in our office. Some of it, if the provider is skilled in that particular area, is very lucrative. The patients much prefer to be seen in our office than to be referred to an unfamiliar office some distance away. (This is called the better-the-devil-you-know syndrome.)

PEER REVIEW

We all are human and fail at times in our "practice" of dentistry. It's still uncomfortable when one of my caring, committed fellow doctors points out a procedural shortcoming to me, or I to him. We do it because of our commitment to our patients and because we know it helps us to grow professionally. Perhaps it shouldn't matter, but knowing my friends and fellow dentists will see those crown margins or endo fills increases my effort to do my best.

As admittedly uncomfortable as it is to have an associate point out a less than perfect result to you, the prospect of a peer review committee or (God forbid) an attorney making the same point is much less appealing.

MUTUAL SUPPORT

"Nobody knows the troubles I've seen"—except another dentist. Staff, a spouse, or a child may be concerned and sympathetic, but no one else knows. It can be a great help to have a friend right in the office who really does understand that at times, even your mightiest efforts aren't good enough.

Emotionally, other doctors have complete empathy, because they have been exactly in your shoes in the past. Physically, they may be able to step in and assist in a clinical situation that is progressing from bad to worse, despite all your efforts. What we do for a living is lonely work. It helps to have a friend close at hand. This friend is not only committed to you emotionally, but your futures are tied financially as well. I can't imagine a more committed advocate than your associate.

All this discussion has been pitched to associates and not to partners for the simplest of reasons: I have never had a partner. I never will. No amount of money would ever tempt me to give up control of a practice I have devoted 20 years of my life to developing. I would certainly sell a part of my incorporated office, but never a controlling interest. If your interest lies in partnerships, you need another book.

I don't mean to sound judgmental concerning partners. Partnership may work wonderfully well for some people and in certain situations. I'm a leader. I don't like decisions made in committee. For me, collecting all possible staff input and then deciding for myself what is best is the only system I'll consider.

CONS

On the negative side of group practice, two things are of major concern to me. After years of effort, I fear that for me, these may be problems not to be solved, but to be endured.

LOSS OF SHARED VISION

The larger the group, the harder it is to share a clear purpose or vision. As you know, our office spent a year writing our purpose. This was completed before we became a multiple doctor practice. For years, our purpose was the epicenter of our practice. Personally, it still reflects what gives the practice of dentistry meaning to me. I'm not sure I can say today that all of our staff is committed to this vision.

A plaque with our purpose inscribed on it still hangs on the wall of every room in our office. We still read this document before each staff meeting. I'd dearly love to tell you all of us are committed to it, but sadly, I can't. Of all the problems we'll discuss, this to me is by far the greatest and the one I seem least able to solve. The sense of teamwork gained from common values just isn't as strong. I wish the same process I use to hire my staff would work in hiring an associate, but besides the fact that I get maybe five applicants for the associate's position as opposed to 50 for the staff opening, I have to consider too many other variables.

As the number of people involved in our group grows, it seems inevitable that the strength of these values is diminished. We have had doctors in our office that were almost scornful of our creed. At first such an attitude was puzzling to me. Part of the reason they choose to join our office was our success. Our purpose played a critical role in our accomplishments. Now I believe I see that though they admire the success we have had, they are threatened by it too. They have a need to assert their independence. I'm afraid it is all too human to belittle or even attack that which you perceive to be stronger or greater than you.

Logically I feel they should study what we have done and emulate the parts that are consistent with their own values. Realistically, I've never employed an associate doctor who I felt attempted to do this. Of course, none of our beliefs or systems are forced on them. They are free to follow our ways or to create their own. My personal philosophy and experience with life shows me no other possible course of action to follow. I'm sure there exist people clever enough to copy a winning concept. Unfortunately, none of the five associates who have graced our office over the years have truly done so. I believe the need of ego to assert itself when it feels threatened is just too strong. If I were an associate in our practice, possibly I would do the same (but I sure hope not).

LOSS OF CONTROL

Maybe this is part of a loss of vision, but it was very hard for me (and I'm sure as hard for my associates) not to be *the* doctor, not to have all the staff and patients be *mine*. If you have an established practice and want an associate to stay, *you have to give up some control of staff and patients*. You can be the team quarterback, but not the king of the office. I don't believe outstanding doctors would like to work in your office—it must become theirs, too. This can't happen unless they are given the authority to do things on their own. (Refer back to our staff meetings: the principles of ownership are the same.)

As I stated earlier, I want no partners. On the other hand, I allow my associates complete control of their part of our practice, as long as the quality of care we provide to our patients is not compromised. We use only the best dental materials, instruments, and labs. All of the doctors have chosen to copy us in these matters. It is in the hours they work and the methods of interaction with patients and staff they adopt that their individuality is expressed.

All doctors and staff are required to attend and participate in our full-office staff meetings. Most of the doctors have chosen not to participate in a morning clearing with their staff or to review each patient's record before the day begins. I state these things only to give a full and honest report on the status of our office. I neither like or agree with their choices, but in reality, they are just that—their choices.

I think they believe (or hope at least) that great success can be achieved without expending quite the effort we put in. How about you? Is there somewhere you go looking for a free lunch?

OTHER PROBLEMS

The minor frustrations, but ones I feel we can some day control or eliminate, include:

Staff conflict. It's true, as staff increases in size, conflict increases geometrically. Also, cliques start to develop, and sadly, people become loyal to "their" doctor. (Loyalty should be to "our" patients, but it doesn't always work that way.) We work consciously and consistently on communication skills—we always have—and continue to devote 40 minutes of each staff meeting to a communication exercise, but these conflicts continue to be an annoyance.

More frequent mistakes. Job descriptions are less clear due to more people being involved in our projects. Also, with expanded hours, a person who begins a job (like study models or postoperative calls), is not always the one who finishes it. This opens the door for more errors.

Communication lines become more muddled, so lab cases may not be sent promptly, or postop calls aren't made at all. Sometimes the same patient is called twice and given the same message by two staffers. A lot of little oversights and errors occur with our current, multiple front-office people compared to when just one or two staff members performed everything. It is easier for duplication of efforts to occur, such as two people calling the same patient to confirm the next day's appointment. Such complications seem inevitable with more people involved in performing the same tasks.

Equipment breakdowns. Due to expanded use of our facilities, we require more equipment repairs. It's not just the added expense, but not having a piece of equipment available when you need it is frustrating. Also, I get a little annoyed every time "my" chair is repositioned. Instead of everything being set just as I prefer, now constant minute adjustments are needed by each doctor. Occasionally, some needed supplies aren't ordered when they should be, or they aren't t replaced in their correct spot.

I guess the answer to these "little" things is a 4,000-square foot office with nine ops, but that eliminates the reduced overhead that, to me, is the biggest advantage of a group.

Each of you can add other concerns I'm sure, but for me, these have been the major considerations involved in a group practice setting. However, the biggest variable will be your own personality. Do you enjoy working with others? Can you submerge your ego (it won't disappear, but for most of us it can be controlled) for the good of a team? With proper leadership, the financial advantages are great, as I think each year's *Dental Economics* survey comparing solo and group practice finances illustrates.

The pressures of dentistry can be decreased for all the reasons we've discussed. But you'll have to look deep inside yourself to see if these advantages make tolerating the disadvantages worthwhile. I urge you to look carefully before you leap. A group practice started without careful planning can closely resemble a hasty marriage. Remember the old saw, "Marry in haste, repent at leisure."

The economies of scale we discussed also come to play in a satellite office situation, with one small twist: they are reversed. That's right, now fixed overhead increases, and net is diminished. I haven't purchased a satellite office, so these comments are philosophical only and not supported by personal experience. If you are tempted to pursue a second practice location, be sure you understand the overhead concerns we discussed here, because those same principles apply to a satellite. Be very sure before you act, because the "repent at leisure" part applies also. I believe you'll discover it's a whole lot easier to buy a dental practice than it is to sell it.

If you have decided that you are interested in either becoming an associate or adding one to your existing office, how do you proceed to identify viable candidates or offices to select from? Let's go on to the next chapter for some answers.

CHAPTER 16

ASSOCIATE
RECRUITMENT

There may be no more challenging undertaking in dentistry than the establishment and successful continuation of a multidoctor practice. Many complex factors are involved in this undertaking, but none is more critical than the initial choice by both the owner of the established practice and the doctor seeking a practice, as to whom they wish to develop an associate relationship with.

As we have discussed, since 1985 I've brought five associates into our dental practice. After making the initial decision to bring other dentists into our office, I began a search for the proper individuals or organizations to help me identify potential candidates. I still remember my surprise and distress when I realized that there really was no viable entity to help me with this critical task.

It is with this knowledge of the vacuum that exists in neutral parties available to lend unbiased assistance to either the dentists seeking an associate or the doctor in search of the proper opportunity in which to practice the profession that I've recorded my thoughts and experiences on the "recruiting trail." While most of my experience has come as the dentist seeking an associate (except for my original search for a practice in 1974), I believe this information will greatly assist dentists seeking a position by revealing to them where and how established dentists conduct their searches.

Recruitment of an associate is a lengthy, difficult, and expensive proposition both for the established doctor and the potential associate. Before you begin, I'd urge you to be absolutely certain of your commitment to bring someone into your practice. I'd strongly suggest that you fully equip your office—redecorating and augmenting your physical plant in any way possible to make it as attractive as feasible—before you begin to interview candidates.

I realize that changes to office physical plants are an expensive, as well as time-consuming task. The temptation is to wait until the associate is hired before updating and enhancing your office. However, after an associate is in place, the motivation to make these changes and to have everything looking its best just isn't as great.

Some of the work done to make your physical plant appear at the maximum of its potential is needed in any event. The equipment that you add will have value (in added function and as a financial asset, as well as in improving the image of your practice in the eyes of your patients), no matter what results occur in the future. Also, you will be ready to put your associates to work as soon as they are able to join you and not be delayed at a critical juncture by needed office preparations.

Enhancing the decor and equipment of your office in preparation for an additional doctor proves your commitment is sincere to any potential associates. To the best qualified candidates, those you'll have to compete with other offices to hire, a fully equipped and beautiful office is a lot more convincing than someone telling them what he or she *plans* to do. These steps are simply another example of creating reality where before was only your vision.

Before you begin the actual recruitment process, you must clarify your desired future with an associate. Do you wish a long-term commitment? If you seek only temporary assistance, you must plainly tell each candidate. If you aren't candid here, there will be pain and anger later when the truth is revealed.

If you do seek a long-term commitment, your practice should be valued and a *tentative* buy-in contract created before your search process has begun. The tentative buy-in agreement simply establishes that on a mutually selected date in the future, should both parties be in agreement, a permanent buy-in can be entered into. It will also state some of the specifics of the future buy-in agreement, such as what *formula* will be used to value the practice.

I see no way that an exact price can be set on any practice for a sale at some date in the future. It is very possible to agree to a formula that, when the proper and pre-agreed-upon practice numbers are plugged into the mutually accepted formula, will yield a practice value agreeable to both parties at any date of their choosing.

Sadly, potential associations often fail, even when both doctors have been happily working together for some time, when it is realized they disagree on the specific arrangements for buying into the practice. I am aware of two cases where the perception of value of the practice differed by 100% between the owner doctor and the established associate seeking to buy in. Instead of a sale that continued an excellent working relationship and viable business for both, each felt the other party to be grossly unfair. The relationship ended in bitterness, instead of mutual benefit. This occurred after years of working together, and all because no attempt to provisionally agree on a buy-in was arranged at the onset of their relationship. Both felt that it could be "done later, when they were both sure things were working out." Now both parties must start over in their respective searching, hopefully wiser from the experience.

The ADA has a simple booklet, *Successful Valuation of a Dental Practice*, Volume 2, that is very helpful in establishing a method to determine a practice's worth. I've read several books on the subject of practice valuation that were longer and more difficult to comprehend than the ADA's effort, but to me none was as valuable and simple to implement. You'll need professional help from accountants and lawyers, but both the senior dentist and potential associate must personally understand the basics of any buy-in arrangements to assure mutual fair treatment. This step is too critical to be left entirely up to a third party's discretion.

If the parties refuse to do their homework in this critical area and instead trust others to take care of these "details," I can promise them they will rue the day. No longer can dentistry see the world of business as an area where competence is optional to the well-being of a practice. Like it or not (and I know the majority of us don't), the realm of business is essential to our practice's financial viability.

Think of the academic courses you were "forced" to take in order to achieve your goal of a dental degree. None of us loved each and every discipline. We were forced to study subjects we didn't necessarily enjoy because they were essential to the attainment of our ultimate goal. In today's world this accurately describes our need to be aware and concerned about the business of dentistry. Too many forces outside our control, be they IRS, OSHA, or the initials of your choice, have too extensive a control of our futures for us to ignore them. The game of dentistry has changed, and whether you agree or approve of the situations, you'd better get used to playing by the new rules.

As a potential associate, I would hesitate to consider an office that hasn't already been equipped physically in anticipation of my arrival or where no valuation and written buy-in agreement exist, even if I had no plans to buy-in for some years in the future. The chance of your agreement floundering when promised changes in the physical plant aren't forthcoming or when a permanent business agreement is attempted at some later date is just too great.

Now the established doctor is certain he wants to bring in another dentist and has proven this to himself and to a potential associate by fully equipping and enhancing the office. The nature of their commitment to a future associate as either long term or short term in nature has been clarified. (Neither option is good or bad, but it is essential that both parties be clear as to what they seek.) A tentative value for the practice, as well as a tentative buy-in agreement has been established. These documents can't be finalized at this early date, but they can be mutually understood and will act as a framework for a final agreement when both parties are prepared to make this step. The remaining task: how to locate the right individual.

I started my recruitment efforts with an ad in the ADA Journal. This became our major instrument to locate recruits, especially those no longer in dental school. Here is the most recent ad we ran. It's no masterpiece, but we did get excellent responses.

American Dental Association
Classified Advertising Department
Box #B271
211 E. Chicago Avenue
Chicago, Illinois 60611

We have an outstanding opportunity for a full-time Associate with buy-in available. Our staff of nine, five fully equipped and modern operatories, and over 5,000 active patients are waiting. Our 1987 gross was over $470,000. We are located in Keokuk, Iowa, on the banks of the Mississippi—an outdoor- and family-oriented community of 13,000. Immediate patient load and income available.

Please call me at (I placed both by home phone and office numbers).

Obviously this ad is a little dated, but I copied it verbatim as it was placed in 1988 for authenticity's sake.

In this advertisement, I attempted to stress the positive aspects of our office (What a unique concept! I should have gone into marketing.): the size of the practice, our past performance, and our immediate patient load are pointed out. This is to draw a response from as many *qualified candidates* as possible.

The brief description of the community will eliminate those interested in an urban setting, while encouraging those seeking a more pastoral location. The size of the practice will discourage those seeking a quiet, lower pressure situation. My goal with this ad was to maximize responses from candidates with a genuine interest, yet to eliminate those searching for either a quiet office or a big city location, so neither of us would waste time.

At one point I placed ads in the state dental journal too, but if potential candidates received the state journal, they had to be ADA members. I'm sure anyone in search of an associate position would look at the ADA advertising section with its much greater circulation. Since advertising in the state journals seems a duplication, wasted time, and wasted money, I no longer place ads in these publications.

The ADA ad is critical to recruitment, but it takes over 90 days to get an ad placed in the journal. This length of time seems totally unreasonable to me and certainly not the way I'd run a business, if we may consider the ADA as such. I've been an ADA member for 20 years. Of my frustrations with the ADA over the years (and there have been way too many to discuss here), the delay in ad placement is one of the most annoying and least understandable to me.

In the 90-plus days you are forced to wait for the ADA ad to be run, there's lots to do. I have dealt with a number of brokers and professional placement agencies. Mostly I filled out forms and had long phone conversations with them. Eventually I'd find out how many dollars it would cost to use them, and then I'd decide to avail myself of their services only if no other efforts turned up good candidates. I hate to think how I'd feel if associates told me they were leaving after I'd spent thousands of dollars to have some organization identify them for me.

So far I've been able to identify excellent people using the other methods we'll discuss, and I haven't needed the assistance of the brokers or agencies. This has saved me paying them a substantial fee, but more importantly, I've learned a lot by being personally involved in the entire recruiting process. I have no bias against these businesses and no stories of misfortune to impart, but again, if you choose to let others perform a job you may not find appealing, I believe it will cost you in the long run.

By far the next most meaningful source of candidates after the ADA ads are the dental schools. We developed a photo album of our attractive office and sent it, along with a two-page cover letter describing our practice, to every dental college in a 250-mile radius. This mailing was followed up a week later by a phone call from me to each institution. Usually the person the dental college has put in charge of handling this information is a secretary or librarian whose job includes "putting these things out" for the students. It's very sad that after four years of involvement with students, most colleges' commitment to them involves nothing more than having someone "put something out" for the students to peruse.

Despite this limited assistance from the colleges, we've always been contacted by a good number of students. Our album, letter, and personal call to each school not only garners us a greater number of responses, but attracts the interest of the most aggressive and highly qualified applicants.

It seems to me that the students today, at least in our Midwest area, are making their postgraduation commitments very early, often a year before graduation. I applaud this preparation, and I suspect it may be due in large part to their perception that it is difficult to find good opportunities "out there." It is a little frustrating to me, if I would like more immediate help, to find the senior class completely committed by January of their final year. However, my advice to both those looking for and those seeking associate positions is that they must plan well in advance. Never allow something as critical as the search for an associate or for the office position that will be your future to be rushed.

Once contact is established with a student, after you've visited with them and they've seen your office and both parties remain interested, I'd recommend a trip to their school. Get the students' permission to see their grade transcripts (you can't see their grades without their authorization) and visit with some of their instructors. I'd only do this with candidates you're seriously considering, because a whole day is usually involved. However, the depth of commitment you and your associate must make to each other, if a permanent relationship is to happen, makes this time well invested. You may choose to combine this trip with a continuing education opportunity, or if there is an instructor at the potential associate's school you admire, you may be able to arrange some time spent talking with this paragon of academic achievement or perhaps watch them treat patients. There is always more to be learned in our profession.

In our rural area, contact with local and state dental societies has never proven helpful in finding recruits. I'd guess in a metropolitan area this could be extremely helpful, and I'd suggest that you explore this possibility if you live in or near a densely populated area.

I've always contacted our area dental-supply dealers when I'm searching for an associate. They are usually enthusiastic and immediately fill out a form describing the type of situation you have available. I've never had a candidate referred by the supply companies, but contacting and providing them with information is a simple process for which no fee is requested. It was a supply representative that guided me to my first and only practice location.

Using these techniques has always given me an excellent group of candidates to choose from—never less than five. Be patient; applications can trickle in over a six-month period, long after your last recruitment effort took place. Making a choice too quickly could mean you miss an excellent candidate who contacted you later in the process.

When I get together with the candidate I try to be completely frank, telling them *exactly* the type of practice we have and sharing our philosophy. I show our strengths and open all financial records to them, including profit and loss statements and even my tax records if they are interested in such things. Many students have no concept of how to analyze practice financial figures, and spending much time on more than the most cursory of business monitors just confuses them and wastes time. Conversely, a dentist who has run his own practice may ask some very candid and excellent questions based on their review of your financial records.

I also show our office's blemishes and imperfections. My interest has always been for a long-term relationship, and after spending many hours and dollars selecting a candidate, having your new associate leave is very discouraging. I never want an associate's departing to be due to a lack of candor on my part. The relationship between the senior doctor and associate dentist must be a truly win-win one, based on complete honesty. It also does the associate no good to mislead the employer doctor concerning his/her qualifications and desires and be awarded the position, only to lose it when all the facts become apparent.

The final selection of the right person for your practice is a completely personal one. Of course, clarifying your values and developing a clear vision of your preferred practice future is essential for any hope of success in this venture. I would recommend a credit check be done on a serious candidate. It is not unusual for a dentist looking for a new opportunity to carry some real financial burdens. I would like to be certain that they have been honest in sharing this information with me, just as I have openly and candidly shared my financial situation with them. You'll need to get the applicant's permission to run this check, but a refusal on their part would afford you a great deal of insight.

Personally checking the references of any potential employee is essential. A few years ago, a physician whose office was next door to mine hired a very attractive young lady to be his office manager. She had previous experience in medical office work. When he finally realized a problem existed, his best estimate was that she had embezzled about $10,000. The frosting on the cake was when he found out she had been fired from two previous jobs for theft. No charges were ever filed in any of the three incidents. I guess this kind of thing could never happen to you? Well, it won't if you check references.

I like to bring the potential associate in to visit when our office is actively treating patients. It is the office atmosphere during these moments, more than any other factor, that *should* help job candidates decide if this is the right opportunity for them. I tell all associate candidates that new patients know if they are in the right place or not within two minutes of first entering our office. The associate candidates should be able to do the same. I suggest that they attempt to suspend their left-hemisphere function for a couple of minutes and get a feel of the office.

When candidates do visit, after being welcomed briefly by me, they are turned over to a staff member for a tour of our office, an introduction to our staff, a cup of coffee, and a quiet visit. We allow the associates to wander about the office after that. I get a lot of insight just by seeing what interests them. My staff is evaluating them during this time too. Of course, they are unaware of this subtle evaluation, and thus more relaxed and candid with staff than they may be with me.

Usually over lunch (for which I have scheduled 90 minutes), our guest and I get our first chance to really visit. I can answer any concerns that may have arisen by now. The type of questions asked is perhaps the most revealing of any single thing in helping me to know this individual.

Some ask repeatedly about job security. Others are fixated on patient load and seek reassurance that they will make money. I have no way of predicting how they will do financially, and I tell them so. I don't know enough about them as dentists to even hazard a guess as to their future performance. We do have, in writing, a copy of how other doctors that have joined our practice in the past have performed financially. I much prefer to provide them with written documents in answer to questions because my memory isn't that great. Also, if in the future a question arises about what was said, we have a common document to refer back to.

After lunch one of my staff gives a guided tour of our community. Again, we are attentive to their interests. In the car with just two people, an even-more-candid conversation often occurs. After this tour, they return to our office and continue to observe (and be observed). At the end of the day we sit in my office for a long talk. Usually by now we both know if this relationship is going to work. Often neither of us is ready to admit it when we feel it won't, but we know.

I answer any questions, ask a few, and try to get a certain feel for our future together. I'll spend whatever time is needed to answer queries and visit, but after an hour or so of one-on-one, both of us usually feel we have enough information.

How we proceed from this point depends on my feelings about our future together. I will certainly reflect on this visit carefully before I reach a decision. I usually have some strong feelings about what our collective future will be before the visit ends. If things seem positive, I may give candidates a copy of our employment contract to study and make arrangements to call in a few days for further discussion. If I am doubtful we have a future, I'll ask them to think our day through and then to get back to me with their thoughts.

Almost always when I feel things won't work, the candidates do too, and I seldom hear from them again.

Developing an associate relationship is a long, difficult job for all parties involved. Certainly whole books couldn't cover every possible consideration inherent in this process. Allow me to sum up my comments:

Both sides must evaluate the situation objectively and be completely frank with each other. Then my advice is simply to choose the individual you *like*. Pick the person you feel good with. After you've narrowed your search to a few qualified candidates, this emotional content far outweighs all the logic, research, and the reasoning you can do. Certainly, do your homework, and after thorough consideration, *hire a friend*.

INVESTMENT STRATEGIES FOR FINANCIAL SUCCESS

CHAPTER 17

CAN DENTISTRY BE A PATH TO FINANCIAL INDEPENDENCE?

I've given it a lot of thought, and I think the problem is they just don't understand. I'm talking about the financial experts who offer all the investment advice. I'm inundated with a myriad of financial data from these advisors. Don't get me wrong, these guys are a lot smarter about money matters than I ever hope to be. It's the *doctor's life* that they can't comprehend. The time demands, as well as the physical and emotional fatigue inheritent in our profession, make a lot of good investment strategies worthless to us.

In my office I go to great lengths to keep it simple. All the advice I need for any given procedure we perform I'd like on a 3" x 5" card. I believe that investing has to be that simplified for most busy practicing dentists to have a chance at financial success.

Does it make sense to you that due to the uniqueness of our professional situation, we should have an investment milieu tailored exactly to our needs? The idea of a need for a different investment philosophy for professionals is one that I have yet to discover in my years of reading business information. Most dentists who get heavily involved in the world of finance and attempt to share their knowledge with their wet-gloved brethren become students of finance and not of dentistry. Soon their expertise leaves the practicing dentist in the dust, confused and uncertain when he/she attempts to follow the learned fellow dentist's advice. These doctors have themselves become investment professionals.

The typical dentist's attitude towards financial matters has always been curious to me. This was especially true in the ancient past when I was a neophyte dentist. The typical dentist I encountered in my salad days appeared, at least at cocktail parties, to be somewhat an expert in matters financial. Why the need to attempt such a facade, I don't know. Certainly we had absolutely no training in this field. Most of us weren't even properly schooled in how to run a dental office, let alone how to invest any surplus funds we might be fortunate enough to acquire. Yet most of my senior-dentist acquaintances in those halcyon days talked knowingly of financial affairs, or so it seemed.

As a result of the articles I have written for *Dental Economics*, I've been involved in many phone calls from dentists all over America who wish to discuss financial matters. These calls have been very candid, unlike the cocktail conversations. Repeatedly I have been informed of the distrust, insecurity, or downright fright (depending on their past investment history) with which these dentists approach the financial and investment world. The cocktail conversation is whistling in the dark, apparently. It seems, as professionals, we feel a need in financial matters to present ourselves as something we are usually not: astute investors.

In these private phone conversations about money, many of the doctors have frightful stories to tell, and I'll scare you in a bit with tales of my own financial misadventures. Some doctors, (perhaps the smarter ones) have become almost paralyzed, unable to move financially for fear of making a mistake. They distrust financial advisers, and intuitively sense they are somewhat at the mercy of this group.

There is real danger inherent in a pretense of financial expertise that is not truly possessed. Of course, when in conversation with someone who actually knows something about the subject of investing, you are seen as a fool. (Remember, it's better to remain silent and be thought a fool, than to speak and remove all doubt.) Sad as such a pretense appears, there exists a true financial risk in such self-delusion: that you actually believe you do understand some of the topics you're discussing and listen to your own advice. Such a blunder could result in severe financial consequences.

What I am proposing here is the development of an investment philosophy, one uniquely suited for each individual dentist/investor. Again, I harken back to clarifying values and interests (pedantic is my middle name). There is no one right way to invest. Below are some generic questions, the answers to which can propel you on your journey to a clarified financial philosophy.

1. How interested in financial matters are you?

2. How difficult do you find investment matters to comprehend?

3. How much time is available for you to devote to financial matters at this point in your life?

4. How much surplus financial resources (that's money) do you have available to invest *right now?* How much do you realistically expect you can save?

These basic questions and many more individual ones must be answered before any possibility exists of coming up with the right financial plan for you. No investment adviser, at any fee, can provide you with the correct answers for your unique situation. No formula can take the place of self-awareness in finance or any other endeavor.

I believe many dentists avoid all study of finance because they feel intimidated and overwhelmed by the vast amount of material available in this field. When they do invest, it is almost impulsively, sort of shutting their eyes, jumping, and hoping all will turn out well. It won't. I want to make you realize that you don't need to know everything about the world of finance to invest in a safe and sane manner. I believe I can provide you with a base of knowledge that will be sufficient to allow you to begin to search for the level of investment expertise that is appropriate for you.

I can do this, not because of my encyclopedic knowledge of the financial marketplace, but because I understand dentists. I know our training, our lifestyles, our time availability, and emotional makeup. I won't suggest a plan that requires an hour a day to use. If you were foolish enough to follow such a plan, in a matter of months it would be abandoned, due to the stress, strain, and time constraints of our profession. What would be the result of the investments made then?

I love to garden. Imagine my garden after several months of diligent work if I totally ignored it for a while. I would have a garden of weeds. Your investment future will be a garden of weeds too, if you invest with sporadic intensity and then find you no longer have the energy, time, or interest to follow up on your efforts, as you must with some investments. We are, beginning at this moment, in the process of designing an investment garden that will be just right for you. Not so large that its care becomes drudgery, yet one that will yield for you the fruits you personally desire.

There are some in our profession who feel very skilled in the world of business and prefer to "swim with the sharks." This section isn't intended for them. It's for us "little fish" in the financial sense. For you superior beings, so astute in financial matters, I wish you luck. I'll also ask you to reflect on the expression used before, to "swim with the sharks." Are you? Is that really where you *want* to be? What is the fate of small fish who due to some self-delusion feel equal to the sharks and take their place among them?

In this financial section of the book, the fields where the fruits of my beloved *net* are invested, we will look at these aspects of the world of investments:

1. What does it take individually to create a situation in which you have the pleasant problem of what to do with your money? In other words, how can *you* save money?

2. We will review the different financial instruments available to begin, or possibly further, your basic understanding of the vocabulary and basic building blocks of information used in this realm. We'll go slowly and define each of the possible investment vehicles I believe are prudent for the majority of professionals to be involved with. We'll also take a brief look at the investment choices that get dentists (and I believe most *everyone else*) in deep financial troubles.

3. I will share with you my own personal opinions, as well as the actual decisions I have made in matters of finance.

How then, does one arrive at the position of having liquid assets available to invest? This destination, much to the surprise of most, is not related to income. I know of people (my parents among them) who were never blessed with great income yet always managed to save. I know many others who have enjoyed incomes well over $100,000 annually for years and have a net worth of negative value.

Your *net worth* is determined by adding all your wealth, or assets, and subtracting all your debt. A negative net worth means your debt exceeds your assets. Debt could be loans, unpaid credit card balances, or any situation where you have an obligation to pay money out. Debt includes mortgages (loans on property, whether home, office, or real estate investments), too. Don't let people tell you they own $1,000,000 worth of real estate without realizing they owe the bank $900,000 on a note. If the value of their real estate drops to $800,000, a not uncommon thing in today's world, does this change in property value have an effect on the bank note? No, the *debt* stays the same. How does their net worth change? From a positive $100,000 to a negative $100,000, because now the debt exceeds the value of the asset. Such is often the fate of "paper" millionaires.

In my office, as I have repeatedly stressed throughout this book, the critical measure of our financial success is *net* (the money remaining after all debt is paid). The vital number isn't production, new patients, or collection percentage—all important figures— but *the* measure I use to judge my success is *net.* In the investment world I look principally at one factor: *net worth!* This is the ultimate measure of financial performance that I observe to determine my financial progress, or lack of same.

Our friends who control $1,000,000 in real estate and have a $900,000 loan have a net worth of $100,000. If they believe their cocktail conversation about "owning" a million dollars in real estate, and worse yet live like they do, they will soon be in financial ruin. *Always* look coldly, yet clearly, at your financial picture. You can lie at parties if you must, but be sure you and your family know the truth. There is a big difference between producing $3,000 of dentistry in a day and having $3,000 to spend. (The final numbers will be just "slightly" altered by overhead and taxes.) Be sure you and your wife both understand this fact.

Before I interrupted myself with the critical message about net worth, I meant to say exactly what you thought: savings and the attainment of a positive net worth are *not related to income.* The equation is very simple. *To have a positive net worth you spend less than you make.*

The opposite (spending more than you take in) gives you a negative net worth. *How much you make has no effect on this equation.*

This makes it tough on the great majority of Americans who haven't saved much, but only because their income, as yet, isn't great enough. They have been waiting for that great day when they would have "enough income to save." They wait impatiently for their "ship to come in," ignoring the fact that they have never even made the effort to create a dock. Rudely, I have removed the level of income as a factor having any effect on savings. But if income doesn't relate to a person's ability to save, then pray tell, what does?

The first and crucial ingredient, vital to building a positive financial future, is *self-discipline.* Most of us couldn't have completed eight or more grinding years of education without possessing a great deal of this character trait. However, when we graduate, we tend to get undisciplined in our spending (we didn't save) and undisciplined in our investments (do it with no master plan, often impulsively).

There is a simple, but inviolate rule you must understand: *Once you spend money you no longer have its use available to you.* For some reason I've never totally understood, most people feel it is easy to spend, but *very hard to save.* Please remember, this is not a truism. We just made up this particular mindset. We can just as easily create a mindset that makes it difficult to spend and easy to save. The relative value of saving or spending is a *decision* we make, not some inviolate truth. The rules and disciplines we use to handle financial matters exist only in our minds, not on a stone tablet brought down from some long-ago mountain top.

In a similar fashion, much of our culture finds it easy to eat and difficult not to. This also isn't absolute truth. It just seems to be the mindset chosen by many people, sometimes to the point of injuring their health. They are free to reverse this mindset. All of us know people who indeed have. We are just as free to choose a lifestyle of saving, or as I prefer to say, of choosing to spend only for things of real value in our lives.

When I left the army and began the practice of dentistry (in that well known hotbed of dental excellence, Keokuk, Iowa) my wife, two children, and I lived in a small two-bedroom apartment. We drove an old car. I paid all my office debt off in March of 1975 (eight months after we had opened the office doors, as you recall from our first chapter). I'd already realized, at the tender age of 28, that money can work against you (as when you pay debt) or for you (when interest is paid to you).

I don't mean to bore you again with my personal financial war stories. I do want you to understand that in the financial arena I have "walked my talk." All the information I'll share with you in the remainder of this book is based on my own personal behavior and not something I think "sounds good." Recall, if it's already been done, chances are it's possible.

You have to decide which it will be for you. If you want money to work for you, then you must get out of debt. (This would be a good time to make a long written list of all the reasons it's *impossible* for you to get out of debt, then decide if you want to finish this chapter.) *Without the self-discipline to get free and stay free of debt, financial independence is almost impossible.*

One thing I never seem to read regarding financial independence: it takes *courage.* Courage to make your own decisions, even if others say you're wrong. Courage not to get a new car, boat, or house simply because someone you know did. Courage to make a decision and commitment to stick with that decision, even when you don't feel like it.

We parents talk with our children about having the strength to resist peer pressure. They don't have to do things simply because "everyone else is doing them." Then we buy the clothes that are at the moment perceived by the majority to be "cool." (Do you really believe hemline length or the width of a tie really says much about you as a person?) We join the right clubs or social groups and esteem a certain group of friends, whose behavior we shamelessly ape. A certain type of car, a certain type of house, certain vacations: all are necessary. If not, we are not true members, and that means we may not belong. True members of a pathetic herd of sheep, of a group of wannabes, whose value depends on the perception of others and ownership of certain possessions, often purchased with money that really can't be spared. Think about this the next time you discuss peer pressure with your children.

There is nothing wrong with following the crowd, as long as that is what you *choose* to do. The danger is when you feel you have to keep up appearances to be accepted. If you carefully make a decision based on a study of your own values, and the choice is to purchase that car, that's fine. If your values say we need to fully fund our retirement plan and set money aside for our kids' education first, then the decision to buy the car because, "Ours is the oldest on the block and what will people think of us if we continue to drive it?" is the act of a moral coward.

Is your family a team? Do you talk about finances? As a leader of this team, have you created a *vision* of what you'd like your collective financial future to be? Or do you pout and feel like nobody understands how tough it is for you when financial decisions go contrary to your wishes? (This last statement is what used to be referred to as fighting over money in our family, before I became an author.) Financially, I couldn't have done much without my wife's understanding and support, but someone on any team has to lead. Often it's the main provider that must supply the vision of financial freedom and constantly reinforce the vision.

The same basic steps are involved in creating a family financial team as went into building our office team. Someone, usually the family member most involved in and knowledgeable about finance, must *create a vision*. This vision must be *shared* with the team, in a way cogent enough that they willingly *adopt it as their own*. If you attempt to force them to follow your vision, constant fighting will ensue. To be a team, your values must coincide. This is especially true of financial matters.

I know a couple well who choose to deal with finances in a codestructive manner. Whatever the husband spends on himself personally, the wife will spend at least as much on herself and vice versa. This pattern doesn't vary even in times when money is "tight." This doubles the impact of unwise expenditures and creates a state of mutual disregard for the *common* financial well-being. Such behavior causes the sacrificing of each other's personal financial well-being, as well as that of the team.

Nothing will yield a return on your investment of dollars and hours like dentistry. Don't spend your time and money on hog belly futures. Did you study bellies (at least those adorning hogs) for all these years? "Dance with who brung you"—dentistry. Use your hours and invest your first dollars there. Don't worry about how to make a fortune in the world of finance. Worry instead about how to have fun and help the people that come to you for care. Do these things in your office, and making money takes care of itself. Never forget, it is the expertise in our profession we rely on to create the wealth we hope to invest wisely.

I have observed a strange behavior pattern that I wish to report to you. I can not really explain it, but will merely describe it. As people develop real financial security, they have a decreasing tendency to spend. Wherever the need to purchase comes from, money in the bank seems to soothe that particular itch. Conversely, the less able one is to afford purchases, the more that "need" to buy seems present. Can you understand buying out of a need to feel "whole," and how real "wholeness" (in a financial sense, at least) might eliminate that need?

Now we'll get to the details of investments—exactly what to invest in and how—but if you haven't bought into self-discipline, a commitment to a financial team (your family and working with them), developing the fortitude to stick with your decisions, investing in your profession, and finding a way to enjoy it, you won't have anything to invest. The little dab of money you'll have will be wasted trying to get rich quick with those hog bellies. Believe me, understanding these concepts and clarifying your values are the critical decisions. After you've accomplished these goals, the attainment of financial freedom is merely a matter of time.

Here is a brief outline of our 3" x 5" simple financial plans. We'll pursue this information in great detail later, so don't be concerned if you feel somewhat lost at this point. This is intended as an overview of our financial game plan only.

STEP 1. This first step brings you to a place where you have something to invest. Remember, these things come *first*.

    a. Work to pay off debt—school, practice, and house. *Compounding* interest will make you rich (if they're paying you) or poor (if you pay them).

        Here's a helpful little hint to aid you in forecasting your progress with either debt reduction or savings. It's called the *Rule of 72*: to find the number of years it will take for debt or savings to double, divide the interest made or paid into 72. (i.e., 9% interest divided into 72. Your money or debt doubles in eight years.) If your debt doubles every eight years (at 9% interest), how can you get out of the hole? Answer: only by getting out of debt.

    b. Set up an emergency fund—a liquid source of assets, containing a sum of money equivalent to at least three months of your normal expenditures. This will give you peace of mind, but also insures you're never forced by a financial emergency to sell your assets when you would prefer not to, and possibly lose capital by this forced sale.

I use a *money market fund* for my emergency fund. This fund should charge no annual fee and allow free checking. Money market funds are safe (no investor has ever lost a dollar in them, to the best of my knowledge), pay a competitive interest rate that rises and falls with short-term interest rates in general, and are completely liquid. (You just write a check to get money from the account.) This is also where you store money that you have available for a short time before spending or investing in a long-term vehicle. We'll discuss money market funds in greater detail later.

c. Start a retirement fund *right away*, not after you're rich. You need time to take advantage of the power of compounding, especially tax-free compounding in a retirement fund.

Let's say you invest $1,000 at age 30 in your retirement fund. This investment comes off the top of your tax dollars (not just a deduction, but as if you were never paid this money. A $100 deduction in a 30% tax bracket saves you $30. But $100 placed in a retirement fund means you pay $0 taxes on that $100.) The money earned in your retirement fund continues to build up tax free until you retire.

Age 30	$ 1,000
38	$ 2,000
46	$ 4,000
54	$ 8,000
62	$16,000
70	$32,000

At 9%, using our Rule of 72 we see that our money will double (compound) every 8 years.

So through the magic of compounding interest, the $1,000 becomes $32,000 at age 70. If you don't begin saving until age 38, you will only have $16,000 available at age 70. This is why an early start to saving is so imperative. Had you been 22 when you invested the $1,000, it would be worth $64,000 at age 70. *Get the most money you can possibly afford into a retirement fund as soon as possible.* The exact type of plan (IRA, Keogh, Corporate, 401-k) is secondary to the need to get money compounding for you. We'll discuss retirement funds later, but try to understand the concept.

Compounding is a key ingredient to financial freedom. If you invest $1,000 in hog bellies at age 30 and lose it all, at age 70, you're out *$32,000*. You've got to understand that *this is the true cost of a poor investment: not just what you've lost, but the loss of the use of the money forever.*

Let's pretend that at the age of 12 I took some of my paper route money (sure wished I had) and placed it in a retirement fund where it earned a tax-free return of 8%. If I added not a penny to that money, but just allowed the interest to compound at that 8%, how much would you estimate to have accumulated in my account when I had attained the age of 76? Would you believe $256,000? All from a single $1,000 investment and the power of compounding. Take one minute and figure it out for yourself. Compounding is the power that can make you rich.

Now, we have these three points because all are critical, but depending on your personal situation you must assign them their priorities. They all must be done, but each of you must figure out for yourself what the sequence will be based on your personal financial situation of the moment.

STEP 2. I use the money I have left after funding a,b, and c to purchase municipal bonds. I prefer not to buy money market municipal bond funds, but the bonds themselves (in $5,000 units). These return tax-free interest—and if you follow my advice you can anticipate "tax problems." (Worse things exist than paying taxes—like having no money.) We'll soon get to a whole chapter devoted to municipal bonds, so allow me to merely whet your appetite with a few tidbits of information here.

When I buy municipal bonds (with my personal money) and government bonds (my retirement fund), I almost always buy whole bonds (I use government bonds in my retirement fund because I don't want to risk retirement money, and these are the safest possible investment). It's tempting to use funds (rather than to buy the bonds themselves), since funds are "professionally managed" (but so are mine—by me— and I don't charge myself a fee to do the managing). But the value of the funds will change daily with fluctuations in interest rates. I'm not smart enough to play interest rates and figure out which way they'll move. When I buy the bonds I never purchase any that will mature in longer than five years. I hold these bonds until they come due and I'm repaid all of my original investment, and then I buy whole bonds again. I'm guaranteed to make the return stated on the coupon of the bond I bought, no matter what interest rates do during the time I hold the bond.

STEP 3. Study the tax codes and keep them holy (i.e., don't cheat). Over one-third of my net dollars goes to taxes, so understanding these laws is imperative. Every couple of years the government changes the rules (i.e., a new "simplified" tax code is adopted). Studying taxes is a part of financial discipline that is unpleasant for me, but it is essential. *If you trust your accountant and lawyer to do your thinking for you, it will cost you!* It's not their money.

I think most doctors intuitively hate anything to do with taxes. *If you wish to be successful financially, you must understand taxes.* Failing to live a tax-wise lifestyle will most likely assure you of never achieving financial independence. Did you get where you are in life by doing things that were easy and that you enjoyed? Well, here's another dirty, thankless job that you *must do!*

I personally know one dentist who has recently declared bankruptcy due to tax problems. I know another dentist who was forced to pay over $100,000 in back taxes, fines, and accountants' and lawyers' fees due to a one-year audit. I also used to be a prison guard. (When you work your way through college, you take whatever job you can get.) No savings of money is worth risking a stay in prison. Trust me on this one. The point: *don't cheat*, even a little, on your taxes. Take every legal deduction allowed. Be as wise as possible in your lifestyle, but don't risk the nightmare that dishonesty on your taxes can lead to.

STEP 4. I've lost money by investing in oil and gas, real estate, and limited partnerships. I haven't lost on puts or calls, commodities, precious metals, gems, or art, only because I've never invested in them. (If you don't understand what these investment opportunities are, be grateful.) I don't play Lotto either. All I know about these topics today is that I don't want to hear a word about them. Dentists work too hard for their money to waste it on poor investments. Stick with quality and compounding interest, two sure things.

It's most important to understand what money is for: not security or happiness, *but to allow freedom and choices.* I choose to practice dentistry 100 days a year. (I like to hunt, fish, garden, play tennis, basketball, read, and lots of other things more than I enjoy fixing teeth.) I've also chosen to go to San Diego, Hawaii, Florida, Breckenridge, and a few times to Chicago and St. Louis in the past year. I've also chosen to spend more time with my family, doing more things to help others, and making an effort to fill my life with joy. Don't lose the focus: money isn't the goal, but it is a key to personal freedom and joy.

I hope this brief financial overview hasn't confused you too badly. I wanted to discuss the most critical area of finance (values, philosophy, etc.), and then do a thumbnail sketch of what we are about to review in great detail in the remainder of the book. If you're a little uncertain as to the specifics of what we discussed, don't be concerned. What is essential at this point is for you to begin to see the critical need for a consistent philosophy about finance and to get a rough idea of some of the material we will now begin to cover in greater depth. I hope you also see how vital these issues are to your well-being and are beginning to believe that finance is an area that, with a little help and study, you can become confident and comfortable with.

CHAPTER 18

HOW TO PURCHASE SECURITIES—MONEY MARKET FUNDS AND CERTIFICATES OF DEPOSIT

Now that we have begun to explore our own personal philosophies regarding investments and at least have looked at the skeleton of a financial plan in a somewhat sequential order, it's time to begin to examine the actual investment instruments themselves. We need a working knowledge of the different vehicles available for investing, as well as some basic information on how and from whom we may purchase the investment instruments we select.

In the preceding chapter I mentioned dentists that I have spoken with concerning financial matters have a general distrust of the financial experts they come in contact with. I mean no disrespect to the members of the august body of financial advisers (I do a little, I guess), but I approach investment advisers as I would a snake I'd found in the woods. The snake is at home in the woods, I'm a visitor. The same is true when you venture into the investment arena. *You* are the neophyte, and you are dealing with professionals. Don't be so arrogant as to think that because it says "Doctor" before your name on the office stationery, you have mysteriously been given insight and powers in the world of finance.

The only appropriate attitude to assume as you begin the process of learning about the world of finance is fear and trembling! *The awareness* of your ignorance is your key to safety. It's been said that those the gods would destroy, first they make proud.

The people who sell the financial instruments you have an interest in purchasing are *professional salesmen.* Make no mistake; selling is their job. For the most part they are well-educated, very informed about their field, and smooth. They create no product. They make their living *taking money* from the people who do produce.

Do you make more income per hour fabricating a three-unit bridge, or performing an exam? Why is there such a disparity? The world of investments has the same inequitable compensation system our industry does.

A broker will make a small, fixed commission selling you a $25,000 government bond, probably less than $100. If he can instead place your $25,000 into a fund his company represents, his commission could be 7% or greater of your total investment dollars. That's a $1,750 increase in his income. It's also a $1,750 decrease in the amount of money you invested. You didn't buy $25,000 of that fund, but only $23,250 after the dealer's commission. If you are sold whole life insurance, his compensation will be quite a bit higher than $1,750. These figures are not an exaggeration. You must understand this when you proceed to buy the safe, conservative investment vehicles I purchase. Each successful bond purchase you make takes a lot of potential income out of a salesman's pocket.

Does it make sense that the salesman will do whatever he can to convince you that safe and conservative is not for a brilliant, and I might add, "happening dude" like you? You're too smart, doctor, to fall for buying bonds. Why lock yourself in to this "modest" return, when stocks, limited partnerships, futures, commodities, and foreign investments offer much greater "potential" returns? The return from such investments is potential for you, as is the possibility of a financial disaster. The only thing guaranteed in this situation is the commission generated to your salesman.

My answer to such jargon from these salesmen, is that I'm too stupid to understand all those diverse products, and too busy to learn all I need to know about them if I could. I also work too hard for my money *and I don't want to lose it.* My first concern with every investment I make isn't the promised rate of return, but *return!* More than anything else, I want to be sure I *get my initially invested money back* from every investment I make.

All the previous statements concerning my lack of intelligence about matters financial, as well as my lack of available time for same, are true. I can't (and don't want to) keep up with the financial marketplace like a professional in the investment industry. I don't have the education, background, interest or time. I also don't have *timely* access to market information. When I receive financial data in Keokuk, Iowa, the information is too dated to be of much use in investment decisions. The Big Guys had this information long ago and have already acted on it. Remember, it's dentistry that got you the money to invest. This is the profession your energies should be primarily focused on. Stick to your knitting! Dance with who brung you! And a couple more cliches I'll spare you.

Remember how the Indian boy discovered the nature of snakes? The reason I remind you of this particular story now is that I want you to remember who you deal with when you buy securities. No matter what they tell you, or how compelling the reasons they give, never forget they are paid on the basis of sales commissions. The nature of this beast is a salesman, no more or less. A fair question to ask is, "What exactly is your commission on this transaction?" Honest men don't fear this question.

Let me add a disclaimer. I'm surely no expert on the financial matters we are about to discuss. But I feel that it is my strength. I'm like you in my background, not like the professional sales people. For my *curriculum vitae*, I'll point to my ability to accumulate wealth. To earn it, save it, invest it, and *not lose it!* I freely admit my ignorance of many of the nuances of finance. My goal is not absolute knowledge of things financial, but rather the accumulation of enough money to make me financially secure for life. That is the goal this information is pitched to, the ability to *maintain wealth while safely increasing it*, not a doctorate in economics.

In the remainder of this book, I will describe some varied types of financial instruments for you. They are instruments in every sense of the word, financial tools (or instruments) to help you perform specific functions. Our task is to help you:

1. *Identify the financial instrument that can best do a* specific *job for you.*

Ever drive a nail with a screwdriver? A screwdriver is a "tool" right? So what's the problem? Wrong tool! Financial instruments work the same way. If you want to set up a fund for your infant's college education, I guess you could do it with one-month CDs (certificates of deposit), just as you could drive a nail with a screwdriver. But before you ruin the nail and screwdriver, look long and hard for a more effective financial tool to perform that particular function.

2. *Learn exactly how and where to purchase the financial instruments you need.*

Where and how to purchase securities seems to be a big stumbling block for a lot of the dentist investors I've spoken with. The obvious way to learn the proper methods to purchase investment vehicles is to ask the people who sell them. There are two problems inherent in this approach.

a. Doctors don't trust these people (as we've discussed).

b. Doctors are loath to appear ignorant, especially in areas where they really *are ignorant* (as they often are in areas of finance).

We'll try to arrange it so you can appear at least half-smart while talking to the financial types, but remember: by comparison you really are ignorant! For your armor when you do battle in the world of finance, you have the knowledge gleaned from nonsales sources (such as myself and some resources I'll suggest) and an abiding belief in your own *lack* of expertise. Never fail to ask a question about an investment because you're embarrassed that you don't understand. Your expertise is in helping your patients achieve and maintain their own optimal level of oral health, not hog bellies.

I'll tell you exactly what I do in all the investment situations we discuss, but please recall how little I know. I don't reveal my investment choices to influence you concerning what is best for you. That depends on your personal investment *philosophy and goals.* You'll also need to have advice from accountants or attorneys about tax matters and to study some of the material I'll suggest before you are ready to begin making your own investment decisions. The accounts of my personal investment decisions are merely meant as one more source of information that may act as a guide on your investment journey. I'll tell you what I do out of a sense of honesty. I'll also explain the errors I've made over the years, egregious and otherwise.

So let's get on to the specifics of the varied investment options that all of us can choose to participate in.

MONEY MARKET FUNDS

We'll discuss this investment vehicle first, because these accounts are the glue that holds my investment strategies together. I currently have 12 of these funds, one in every bank or brokerage house where I conduct any investment activity. Besides my main investment accounts in our office (mostly for retained corporate earnings that we'll discuss later), retirement plan, and personal investments, we also have money market accounts for each of my four kids' UGMA (defined later), a separate one for my wife's earnings (we have "her" savings and "our" savings), one each for my wife's and my own IRAs, and two others with local brokers. I use these accounts to store cash while I'm waiting for investment opportunities and to hold amounts of money too small to be placed in longer term investments.

Money market funds are very easy and simple to open. All banks and brokerage houses have them available. They require nothing more to open such an account than filling out a small one-page form, similar to what is needed to open a checking account. Usually the minimum balance is very small, often as low as $100.

These accounts are completely *liquid.* That is a key word in our financial vocabulary. The easier it is to get money out of your investment vehicle, the more liquid your investment is. If you have a five-dollar bill in your hand, that's real liquid. If you have money in a fund that penalized you for early withdrawal (many mutual funds and CDs do), that is highly illiquid. *Every* investment has some degree of liquidity. It is neither good nor bad. If you wish to place money in a situation where you have easy access to the funds at any time, you will desire an investment with liquidity. If you're positive you won't need the money, can gain a better yield by investing for a longer time frame, and can "lock in" that yield, you would choose illiquidity.

Cash is most liquid; checking accounts with no fees and unlimited free check writing (i.e., no barriers to removing money) are almost as good, as are the money market funds we're currently discussing. Most real estate is very illiquid (please see the chapter on investment losses I have known).

Money market funds are collections of short-term assets bought in large units (often millions of dollars) by the big companies who create the funds to give the fund the maximum possible yield. (Financial institutions will pay a higher rate of return to someone who loans them a million dollars than they will to someone who loans them a thousand. It's simpler and cheaper for them to process the big loans, and this reduction in their effort and expense justifies a larger yield.)

The investments made by the funds themselves are short term in nature. Information concerning the average length of time money in the fund is invested for is always available, as is the current yield the fund pays, by asking the manager of the fund or by looking this information up in investment publications such as *Barron's*. The fund's average length of investment is usually from 30 to 60 days. The fact that their money is tied up for such a short time is what makes these investments so liquid. They will have assets maturing daily, so they can easily pay money out promptly to any member of their fund who desires it.

There are usually no fees to open these accounts, and most of them have almost unlimited free checking. A big advantage of these funds for investors is that money can be placed automatically into them from returns earned on other investments, so interest isn't lost while checks are "in the mail."

Let's assume you own some bonds that pay interest every six months. A computer in the bank or brokerage house that holds your investment "sweeps" money into the money market account daily. This means when the interest check from your bond is issued, the company that holds your account will place the check in your money market fund the same day it is paid, so you begin earning interest immediately.

Another way to handle this situation is to have the check mailed to you, hang it on the refrigerator for x days, then mail it into an interest-yielding account. When the check finally gets there it will begin to earn interest, assuming you don't lose the check somewhere in the handling process.

Big deal you say, a couple of days' earning interest. You will be making investments for the rest of your life. Besides the loss of interest income caused by the delay in getting the money to an interest-paying account, you'll lose checks in the mail (or on the refrig). Just handling the money, even if you do no more than place it in an envelope, stamp, and mail it, is a hassle, as well as a possible source of error and confusion.

This system, employing money market accounts which automatically sweep and deposit all monies daily, is the best in total return (no lost time or interest) and the safest (no lost checks). Maybe most importantly, it sets up a *system* that runs itself automatically. As your investments grow and interest checks become common, the inconvenience of handling them increases. It's much more efficient to set up a system that automatically reinvests from your first investment.

How safe are these highly liquid funds? Good question. As we discussed last chapter, to the best of my knowledge, no one has ever lost a penny in money market funds. If you are really safety conscious, there are many of these funds that buy only U.S. government bonds. That's as safe as it gets, unless God will invest your money. The return on funds investing in only government bonds will usually be a fraction of a percent point less than the interest paid by "normal" funds that loan to banks and industries. There are also money market funds investing in only municipal bonds. Their interest income will be federal-tax free.

The choice of regular, government, or tax-free money market funds depends entirely on which gives you the greatest after-tax yield. Most funds will let you transfer money between the regular, government, and municipal funds at no charge. You just call or write and request whatever money you choose be transferred to the fund you prefer at the moment.

I usually use the regular funds (not government) because the majority of the time they generate a slightly higher yield. I don't leave much money in these accounts. This is where money builds up until I have saved enough to make a longer term investment. With these funds, I'm not too worried about safety, due to these funds' excellent history of no defaults and the relatively modest amounts of money I keep in them.

I have these accounts *everywhere I have an investment*. I like the convenience of the money the investment returns being invested immediately for me, and I like the extra dollars of interest I earn. Over a lifetime, if you develop significant savings, the total dollars saved by the instant reinvestment of capital will be substantial.

CERTIFICATES OF DEPOSIT

Better known as CDs, this is money you loan to a bank. I don't like or trust banks as investment entities. It's nothing personal (some of my best friends are bankers, and if forced to admit it, I even have a lawyer friend or two). What frustrates me is that I have no accurate or simple way to judge the stability of a bank. I also don't know where the money I put in a bank is going to finally be invested.

If I put money in a CD from a local bank, it may loan it to Argentina for all I know. You get an excellent rate of return, at least on paper, from loaning your money to Argentina. This outstanding return makes the bank's balance sheet look good. The problem is Argentina has a bad habit of not paying its loans back.

My major concern with loans to banks is that a lot of banks and savings and loans have gone broke in the last few years. I know the government insures them, and so far everyone has gotten at least most of their investment back. Of course, you may have to wait months to get the use of your money back, and you may receive no interest during that time, but I'm pretty sure that if you stay below the $100,000 FDIC and FSLIC insurance limit, they'll return your money some day.

My question is, Why take the risk? The yield on CDs is usually pretty close to government bond yields. (Quick now, what does it tell you if the yield is a lot higher? Additional risk, right?)

You can purchase CDs from banks, S & Ls (savings and loans), or the brokers that sell you bonds and stocks. I guess, consistent with my philosophy, I don't want a tiny difference in yield to threaten my return of capital. I'll just buy government bonds instead.

When you purchase a CD, you pay only a small commission. They are backed by the U.S. government up to $100,000 per institution. (Maybe the government has needed to do too much backing the last few years to make me happy.) You get no tax deduction or any tax break on the interest CDs pay (Government bonds are free of state and local tax, and municipal bonds are free of federal taxes, and sometimes state and local tax too, as we'll see later.). Of course, on *any investment* you place in a qualified retirement plan, the interest it generates is tax free.

Dentists frequently purchase CDs, because they are simple to understand and to buy. They also make your friendly local banker happy. They are perceived to be a very safe, if relatively low-yielding investment. I am trying my best to give you unbiased financial information. My feelings about CDs may be based more on "emotions," than on completely objective criteria. I have purchased CDs and never suffered a loss or experienced any kind of problem. I have also never been bitten by a rattlesnake. It may be unfair of me, but I don't *ever* play with rattlesnakes, and I almost never purchase CDs.

Let's go on to study some financial instruments that over the years have been more to my favor.

CHAPTER 19

STOCKS— CONFESSIONS OF A BOND MAN

I've heard that the act of confession is good for the soul. Mine could use any and all possible help, so I would like to publicly admit in this forum that for the majority of my adult life I have been a bond investor.

Truly, you may say, a venial sin, at worst. I'm not sure you'll still think so after all the gruesome facts have been revealed. Allow me to begin my act of contrition.

As I have related to you, dentistry has rewarded me kindly, at least in a financial sense. Despite my addiction to bonds, at age 46, I have an annual income from investments in excess of $86,000 per annum. I state this in no way to mitigate my culpability, but simply to be complete in all the facts. If anything I feel worse about my bond addiction, because I was given fiscal opportunities to do so much more. In Luke 12:48, the Scriptures say, "From everyone to whom much has been given, much will be required" (New Revised Standard version).

Many would wish to be guilty of an offense punishable by an $86,000 per year return. But you see, mine is a sin of omission, not commission. Let me state some facts to further aid in clarifying the issue:

FACT 1. Historically bond yields have about equaled the rate of inflation, while stocks have returned a yield 5%–6% *above* the inflation rate.

FACT 2. Over the last 70 years the average annual yield from investments made in stocks has been 10.3%. For the same 70-year period, the yield from bonds has been 4.8%, or less than half the return stocks have averaged. Using our Rule of 72, we see that investments will double every 7 years on the average 10.3% stock return and double every 15 years by the 4.8% bond pay out. This is of little real significance to investors—if they are going to live for 700 years.

FACT 3. According to the Ibbotson SBBI Yearbook (whose function it is to keep track of such mundane things), over the last 64 years, $100,000 invested in bonds would have yielded $1,600,000 today. The same $100,000 invested in stocks would be worth $25,500,000.

FACT 4. (The *piece de resistance* and chief etiology of my distress and pain.)

a. One thousand dollars invested in the S&P 500 on January 31, 1940 would be worth $333,371 today. (Standard and Poor's 500 is the average value of 500 of the stocks from the largest companies being traded on the exchanges and is used as a sort of barometer of overall stock performance. The more commonly quoted Dow Jones Industrial Average includes only 30 stocks in its computations.)

b. If you added $1,000 each year to the initial $1,000 investment, you would have a portfolio worth $3,554,227 today from your $52,000 total contributions.

c. If you had added another $1,000 each time the market average *dropped 10% in a year,* bringing our total investment to $83,000, your portfolio would now be worth a not-inconsiderable $6,295,000.

These results are derived from the *market average* for these periods. They are not based on some hot-stock picking ability. There are any number of mutual funds available today which, through the magic of computers, automatically adjust their portfolios to yield a return equal to this S&P average. These instruments are called Index Funds. Today anyone can easily and predictably guarantee their return to equal the S&P 500 average, simply by investing in the afore-named Index Funds.

Now, even for those wealthy doctors who are hard to impress, an $83,000 investment yielding $6,295,000 is noteworthy. You do that a few times, and you're starting to talk some real money!

Do you understand my consternation? These numbers are public knowledge, available to anyone. I have always favored bonds—muni, government, corporate—I knew no shame. It is true, I have always had a part of my portfolio in stocks, but only with utility companies, and then never much more than 15% of my total investments was entrusted to these instruments. If anything, had I been paying attention at all, this dabbling in stocks should have shown me the error of my ways much earlier, because my own stock's yields have greatly out-performed my bond investments over the years.

When various and sundry forces lead me to discover these facts, I felt confession was my only hope. As for my poor bonds, I believe one other tidbit of information will suffice to put them in their proper place. It deals with the ugliest investment force of them all: *inflation*.

FACT 5. An investment of $100,000 in a 30-year bond in 1962 would have a purchasing power of $33,000 when it matured in 1992, in terms of 1962 dollars. (Maybe I should offer a course for the investing dentist: How to Create a Million Dollars with Bond Investments: first, start with $3,000,000; and then just wait 30 years.)

HOW I BECAME A STOCK INVESTOR

Let me recount for you the sorry tale of how I was torn from the pastoral bliss and serenity that my life as a bond investor had been by the rude awakening of what potential investment returns I had been missing. It started innocently enough with a course given last December in Chicago. Now, I attend a lot of continuing education courses. Most of them are safe enough, so I had no idea of the cruel fate awaiting me at this meeting.

The course dealt with investments. It was an area of study I had ignored for long years in my hubris. I felt erudite and sophisticated in this arena. The course was presented by Sarner, Collier, and Associates and lead by the distinguished and droll Richard Collier himself, along with a small host of luminaries from the financial community. The course was packed with dentists eager to improve their investment skills. After two days I had the disquieting feeling that an erudition scale of the course attendees would have found me in the lowest quadrille.

The information thrust upon me during this course set me off on an odyssey of exploration into the financial marketplace. Quite a few books, journals, and long hours of diligent studies later I stand before you, a man repentant.

From my studies I must note three extraordinary resources. They are the two recent best sellers by Peter Lynch, recently retired head of the legendary Fidelity Magellan Fund, entitled: *One Up On Wall Street* and the more recent *Beating the Street*. (These worthy tomes are available in any book store and are enjoyable reading, even for those as ignorant of the nuances of stocks as I.) Most of the woeful statistics concerning bond and stock yield comparisons were borrowed from the works of Messrs. Lynch and Collier. A trial subscription to a stock information service called Value Line has also been instrumental in my metamorphism. You may receive information about Value Line by calling 212-687-3965 and speaking with a computer.

I have asked myself why I kept my head firmly in the sand and ignored equities for so long. I like to flatter myself with the idea that I am bright enough to note the obvious. The answer isn't one I'd prefer, but I believe my recalcitrance was mostly due to fear. I was afraid I would lose money in the market. Due to the evils of inflation, there is no reason to fear losing in the bond market. Given time, it's a sure thing. I believe laziness played a part too. I have labored long and hard for four months investigating equities, and I know I have only scratched the surface of all the information available. Lest this ugly specter of hard labor daunt you, please return for a moment to the facts on yields from stocks listed above.

Wherever my deepest resistance came from, its effects are persuasive to the general public as well. In 1990 only 17% of household investments were in stocks. Of the 3,565 mutual funds that were extant in 1992 (that is an accurate figure which grows daily), only 25% of their capital was invested in stocks.

I don't currently own mutual funds. I have gone cold turkey from bonds to buying stocks directly. I'll pass on a few more sources of information on the markets that have been of great help to me. I have neither the expertise nor the space to discuss specific stock selection methods with you in this forum. I will relate two facts: Of the mutual funds that invest in stocks, about 75% of them annually *underperform* the market average. Said another way, if you invest in the Index Funds we discussed, you can be assured of an average return in the top 25% of all stock mutual funds in existence.

As for the bond funds, basically *all of them underperform* the bond market average. This shocking fact (to me at least) is because bond funds all select from the same pool or menu of bonds from which you and I can choose. From the yield of these bonds the fund managers deduct their fees and expenses. These costs reduce the fund's return to a point below the natural (coupon) yield the bonds they purchase pay out.

Two valuable sources of investment help I have identified are:

1. The National Association of Investors (313-543-0612) and

2. The American Association of Individual Investors (312-280-0170).

Both associations offer for a modest annual fee, unbiased assistance (neither sells anything but information) to individuals who desire to invest wisely.

To help assuage your fears of losing money, let me point out that there have been in the history of the market 40 declines of over 10% and 13 over 33%. The market has recovered from each of them. The secret is understanding the long-range picture and not selling in these times of market distress. As Peter Lynch so eloquently states, "It's not the head, but the stomach that determines the fate of stock pickers." Proper *diversification* (what my grandma called "not putting all your eggs in one basket"), owning a minimum of five quality stocks, and a *long-term (five years minimum) focus* on stock investments greatly reduces your risk in the market.

Because these two points are so salient to your financial well-being, I ask your permission to wax pedantic: to prosper in the market you must diversify by investing in at least five companies, and you must *stay in the market long term*. These two factors greatly reduce the risk that all readers of this book know accompanies greater rewards.

As to the exact form this moment of epiphany has manifested itself in my personal investments, I am studying the market and despite the current inflated prices, finding a few stocks I like. As my bonds mature, I am investing that money in stocks. I feel no need to liquidate my existing investments in bonds, especially with such an expensive (at least in historical terms) stock market to select from. You could say I am making the transition to stocks through a natural attrition of bonds.

Once again, I urge you to save. It is the path to freedom and the only honorable way to live. Debt is a form of slavery which people choose when they purchase things they have not as yet earned the right to possess. As doctors we have the education and financial ability to elect a better fate.

As to the many voices extolling bonds, it is the investment of choice for those (as was I) too uninformed, too apprehensive, or for whatever reasons, prefer not to purchase equities. Bonds are still a valuable and essential part of any investment plan, and we'll discuss them at great length in the chapters that follow.

If you are tempted by the greater rewards stocks offer, you must *turn off the TV*. You may choose to begin your education with some of the resources I've listed here. Perhaps a successful fellow dentist you admire would agree to become your mentor on investment matters. There is no problem finding information to begin your stock education. The quintessential ingredient is the *desire* to achieve financial independence.

Remember all you sacrificed to get your dental degree and establish your practice? Now to thrive financially you must give up more of your time and labor. Compared to a year of professional school, however, the price required is quite inexpensive. It saddens me to visit with so many doctors who have the ability to excel financially, yet are struggling so in this arena.

Only study and earnest labor will enable you to garner the potential rewards that stock investing offers. This is not an activity suited for a dilettante! You can't be a successful stock investor if you only pay intermittent attention to the market. You must pay the price of perpetual diligence if you wish to achieve the higher yields equities promise. You can no more expect to succeed in the art of investing without acquiring the needed knowledge than you could expect someone to learn dentistry in a weekend.

Again I must ask that you clarify your values as regards investments. Do you have the desire, time, and energy to undertake the efforts successful stock investing demands? There are many alternatives to stocks we will soon discuss, but in the long run none offers the historic yield of stocks. However, none of the alternative investments require the knowledge, persistence, and dedication that investments in stocks do. If you begin to invest in stocks, then lose interest, you'll lose money. What has been your past pattern towards commitments in general and investments in particular? You have the ability to do well in stock market investing. Do you have the energy and desire? Only with clear values can you answer that question, and for your financial success the correct answer is critical!

If you feel like buying stock on a hunch or tip, do yourself a favor and send the money to me or donate it to a charity. The resultant loss of capital will be less painful. Discipline and consistent effort are required to succeed in this venue. If you *choose* to exercise neither, better stick to lotto as your best chance at the American dream.

Since you've survived the fierce winds of hyperbole that have buffeted you so far concerning investments in equities, let's allow ourselves a few calmer moments to consider some of the more mundane factual matters concerning stock investments.

The act of purchasing stocks is fairly simple. You can buy them from big national brokerage houses such as Merrill Lynch or Dean Witter. There are also discount national firms like Charles Schwab where the commission you pay to purchase the stocks you select is smaller, but less information and assistance are offered. Local and regional brokerage houses will also gladly handle your transactions. For the last several years banks and savings and loans have been able to sell stocks too. All of these sources will be happy to provide you with the money market swept accounts we have discussed earlier for your investment convenience.

Stocks of larger companies, those listed on the New York and American Stock Exchanges, can be purchased at the same price on any given day from all of the previously named sources. If you buy a share of AT&T on July first, you will pay the same price, except for variation in sales commission, no matter which of the sources you choose to make your purchase from.

Stocks of small companies not listed on the exchange will exhibit a lot more variation in the price you pay when you purchase them. If you choose to invest in these small companies, the potential rewards are much greater. *So are the risks!* You'll need to do a lot more homework before you're ready to invest in these smaller corporations.

So which of the above listed sources is the best to purchase stocks from? Depends. If you need a lot of help and advice, the big national firms can supply it. If you do your own thinking and don't want to listen to the sales pitch of brokers (always remember the nature of the beast), a discount broker will handle your transactions for a much smaller fee, as well as reduced conversation.

Perhaps the most critical factor in your decision about where to purchase equities is finding a broker that you personally feel comfortable with. This is no mean feat. Consider how many relationships you were involved in before you selected a spouse (and even then it may not have turned out that well).

What do you seek from a broker? It depends on your values and interests. Honesty and a commitment to listen and answer the questions I ask (as opposed to selling a product of their choosing) are essential to me.

Also, no broker is an expert on every conceivable investment vehicle, so as you refine the investment areas that interest you, such as utilities, growth stocks, small caps, or others, you'll need to discover someone with expertise in these specific areas.

The only method I am aware of to identify the critical right broker for you is trial and error. I wouldn't consider selecting any broker until I'd talked at length with several representatives of their profession. Remember how much effort we put into office team selection? Well, the broker you pick to work with you is also a vital team member. The selection process should be lengthy and diligent. Over the years, as you mature and your investment objectives do too, changes in your team will be needed. The right broker can be a tremendous asset to you in investing. The wrong choice can also seriously damage your chances of financial success.

Brokers are not there to make investment decisions for you. I have never purchased any investment only because some "expert" suggested I should. Brokers are there to supply you with information and feedback. Then, when *you have made your decision,* they will execute the trade you order. No broker knows you, your financial and emotional makeup, or your values well enough to make the best possible decisions for you.

The information available concerning equities is overwhelming. The sources I have listed earlier will keep you busy studying for months. Allow me to add one last addendum to this process.

There are many types of stock in thousands of companies. The risks and possible rewards cover the entire spectrum of investment possibilities, from a complete loss of every dollar you have invested when a company goes bankrupt to a 1,000% return possible if you can select a young Wal-Mart. In the following chapter, we'll look at one type of stock investment I have used: utilities. These companies are historically steady, slow growing, and dependable. They pay a good dividend, usually very competitive to a similar quality bond's yield. For retirement funds, the kids' college funds (UGMA as discussed in Chapter 23), or the retained corporate earnings of the next chapter, these are my investments of choice.

In the afore-named situations, you want stability and steady growth. You want to avoid at all costs a loss of principal, but instead to enjoy the growth of tax-free compounding that all of these situations offer. If you are conservative in nature, near retirement, or just don't want to work hard to understand and to follow stocks, utility stocks are an excellent investment choice for you.

There exists a whole universe of stocks outside the shallow orbit of the high-dividend, low-growth utility stock galaxy we have just visited. The sources I have listed for your study will guide you as you begin your exploration of this world, should you be so inclined.

Over time your investment in high-quality, high-dividend stocks (such as, but not limited to, utilities) should yield you a minimum return of 10%–15% a year. If you decide to stray into the more daring and unexplored parts of the stock universe, be vigilant. You will need to work much harder to comprehend this broader universe. You can experience both greater growth and larger losses here. Please remember the old maxim from poker, and in this higher risk arena, don't play with money you can't afford to lose.

CHAPTER 20

CORPORATE
RETAINED EARNINGS
(The "Secret" Benefit)

To incorporate or not to incorporate: that is the question (my apologies to Mr. Shakespeare). In the 20-plus years I've been a practicing dentist, the questions concerning the efficacy of the professional corporation (P.C.) form of practice structure continues to be a subject of debate within our profession. Much as with our old board exams, the question stays the same, but the correct answer keeps changing. Such vagaries in fashion as concerns the pros and cons of incorporating dental practices can be attributed to our ever-changing tax codes, since it is the degree of tax advantage (or lack of same) that is the central issue in any discussion regarding professional incorporation.

In 1976, when I incorporated my practice, it was a slam-dunk decision. If you had even a moderately successful practice, the advantages of the corporate structure far outweighed any negative considerations. As the years and the tax codes waxed and waned, the issue has become far from clear-cut. While we have gone through periods of decreasing interest in corporation status, today's business climate seems to once again be swinging in favor of professional corporate status.

According to the 1991 ADA Survey of Dental Practice, 28% of general practitioners and 52% of dental specialists practice in corporations. This works out to an overall 31% of dentists who are incorporated.

The incomes of these corporate entities also tend, on average, to be higher than that of their nonincorporated brethren. Again referring to the ADA Survey, the mean income of unincorporated dentists was $215,240, as compared with a mean income of $319,170 for those in a corporation. I have some strong opinions why this disparity would be large, but that is a complex subject and best left for another time and place.

I have read several recent dissertations concerning the advantages of incorporation. These accounts seem to dwell on two features. First, corporate status leads to a forced compliance to a set of standards the corporation structure demands, thus creating a more disciplined structure for we somewhat undisciplined dentists to work in. Secondly, there exists for corporations what seems to me some rather minor financial advantages of paying for life and disability insurance with before-tax dollars.

Both of these benefits exist, and the advantages they give to the practitioner are substantial, yet there remains one advantage to corporate status that I have searched for in vain in the printed media. I believe today this facet of incorporation to be more timely than ever. It dwarfs the other perquisites of corporate identity in its effect on my favorite statistic of them all: *net personal worth.*

But before revealing my little "secret," I need to share a bit more background information to help our understanding of this issue.

The same laws that have so attenuated the benefits of corporate status have crippled the effectiveness of pension plans. Most of the financial benefits of IRAs have been taken away from us because we are not granted a tax deduction for our contribution if our adjusted gross income exceeds $35,000 for a single or head of a household or $50,000 for a married couple filing jointly. Nondeductible or voluntary IRAs are allowed, but these require the use of after-tax dollars for their source of contributions and thus are of little benefit as pertains to tax savings. (Why does our government structure continue to punish people who save? Could it be simple envy?)

In the realm of business retirement plans, laws that were established theoretically to help improve coverage for employees by widening the parameters of who, when, and at what percentage staff members must be covered have made pension plans a losing proposition for the doctor/small business owner who must fund them. I have been told by the ubiquitous "experts" that if 70% – 80% of the money placed in a retirement plan doesn't go to the doctor, the plan doesn't make sense for the doctor financially. I doubt there are many retirement plans extant, given today's tax statutes, which will allow the doctor that level of personal contribution.

There still exist intrinsic reasons to have a retirement plan for your office. You may be committed to your staff's personal and financial well-being, or you may feel offering such a plan promotes job longevity. (You could also be afraid of what your staff will do to you if you quit funding now.)

All these reasons are fine ones to keep a plan intact, but wouldn't it be nice to be able to put money away, tax free, *just for you!* That would seem to be at worst a venial sin. It was you who earned a degree and then took the investment risk in establishing your own business. Your name is on the bank note; the legal liabilities and obligations that accompany our chosen profession fall squarely on your shoulders alone. Why shouldn't you receive more of the reward for what is mostly your creation?

Good news! For incorporated doctors such a thing is possible. This plan requires *no expense to set up or to run,* not even any additional forms that must be filled out.

At long last, it's time to reveal the secret we've hinted at so broadly: *retained corporate earnings.*

Retained earnings are simply profits that are not removed from the corporation. Each corporation is allowed to keep some of its own profits, but the totals retained must not exceed a $150,000 limit, or some extremely stiff tax penalties will be inflicted by your favorite Uncle Sam. You may not be aware of this corporate benefit, but Uncle is, and he has his eyes on you.

Big deal. Leave the money in the corporation. So what? It has to come out some day, and what about the dreaded "double taxation" of corporate assets? These are good questions to which I would respond:

1. The money retained (i.e., profits not paid out) by the corporation can be invested in stocks of U.S. corporations that pay a dividend. *Seventy percent of the dividends paid out to stocks held*

in another corporation is free of any tax (known more formally as the corporate dividend exclusion). Interest payments have no such tax exclusion, so be sure your corporate investments are in dividend-paying assets. The remaining 30% of the profits you earn are taxable at the corporate rate (34% as of this writing), but we'll illustrate how to deal with the conundrum shortly.

2. My corporation has never paid any taxes. I hope no dentist who is both incorporated and conscious has. Before the corporate year ends, any profits are simply paid out in salary. This choice (called a timely election in tax talk) eliminates any corporate tax. But due to business expenses and *depreciation*, not all the money you earn must come out of the corporation to avoid corporate taxes. My P.C. (Personal Corporation) has thousands of dollars in tax losses to "carry forward" into future years. These losses, mostly from depreciation of major equipment purchases, *shelter the dividend income our retained earnings stock produce from any tax.*

Depreciation schedules, as with all tax laws, have changed over the years. Here is a quick cursory review of the most commonly depreciated items in dental offices, again as of this writing. Computers, telephone systems, and cars are depreciated over a five-year period. Dental equipment (units, X-rays, etc.) has a seven-year depreciable life, and buildings are depreciated over 30½ years. These dollars of depreciation shelter profits from corporate tax, and thus allow the taxable 30% of your retained earning to go tax free.

Let me amend my last statement. I'm not sure anything is allowed to remain tax free (and if it is, I'd guess that oversight will soon be corrected by our voracious government and its deficit). Some day taxes will be paid, so the correct sobriquet is tax deferred. When will these taxes be paid? Whenever *you* decide to remove the money from the corporation.

That could be as you near retirement, and your income tax level decreases. It could be when you choose to pay for your new home. (There exists no law that you *must* have a mortgage. Remember, I never did.) It may be when you choose to purchase a needed addition to your office armamentarium. It could be when personal tax rates go down. (Mr. Reagan lowered taxes, and these things do tend to cycle. We're just in the unpleasant part of the cycle at the moment. Taxes really could go down. At least, since it's happened before, I believe it's possible.)

I've used some of my retained earnings to purchase a nine-terminal computer system and also to remodel and to enlarge our office. Both of these investments generated further depreciation dollars, thus allowing more tax-free retained earnings. Also, it's nice to have the ability to pay cash for such things, if you choose. I don't miss dealing with bankers or paying them interest.

My main point is that the timing and purpose to which these dollars are used is up to you. In the interim, the dividends paid by these stocks are compounding tax free. If well-chosen, the value of the stock you selected is also increasing with time.

Let's review our plan quickly. We have identified a system that enables incorporated doctors to *invest with before-tax dollars* as well as allowing the *dividends they pay to compound tax free*. We don't have to pay any expenses to set up or to manage our plan. The money is shared with no one (except, of course, your spouse who will probably get it all some day anyway). You have *complete control* over how and when it is invested and also when you choose to withdraw the money and use it.

To take advantage of this or any other investment plan, you must save! But this is money neither you or your family will see, because it never leaves the corporation as salary (and thus is never exposed to personal income tax). There will be not only no temptation to spend it, but since the money stays in the corporation, no possible (legal) way to spend it for personal use. Because neither the money nor the interest on it is ever taxed, it builds up much faster than personal savings (made up of after tax-invested dollars and taxed returns) could ever possibly match.

I have chosen to invest my corporation's retained earnings in utility stocks. Utilities pay a high dividend and are a legal monopoly, so there is little danger of them going out of business (be awfully hard to run a handpiece if the power companies shut down). Since I expect these investments to remain in the same stock for years, I buy the highest quality of utility stock. I'll share with you a quick and easy way to tell which utility stocks are high quality. They have *lower dividend yields*.

Don't be facile in the use of retained earnings and then be a pig for high yields. High yield in any investment is caused by higher risk. (Where have I heard that before?) I don't want to follow these stocks more closely than to check on their prices once a month. I have enough things to worry about. This money is compounding tax free. We take no chances when investing this type of asset. Given time, the power of compounding in this tax-deferred situation will make us rich, if we don't lose some of our savings due to poor investment choices.

There have been many studies to illustrate the fact that over the long haul (five or more years), higher quality stocks out-perform higher yielding equities in total return. This is because the higher quality stocks increase in price more quickly as the companies issuing the stock experiences superior growth compared to weaker utilities. Outstanding companies also raise their dividends more frequently and by a greater amount. You don't have to fear a reduction in dividends from quality companies, either. With just a little research, you can find a group of companies to select from who have raised their dividends at least 10 years consecutively and have never missed a dividend payment. Any competent stock broker can provide you with such a list, but you will learn more if you do your own research. These stocks are the prudent dentist's quarry for retained earning investments.

Selection of stocks is a complex, multifaceted issue. It will require careful consideration on your part. Again let me stress this point. If you choose to save in your corporation and invest in dividend-bearing stocks such as utilities, do the unnatural thing and take a lower yield. Do you believe companies pay a higher return because they like you? Reward equals risk. If you do lose (heaven forbid) principal, the loss can be used against (or to offset) corporate profits. (Losses can't be used to reduce taxes in a retirement plan investment, because there is no tax to reduce.) But quality investing in a diversified mix of a minimum of five high-quality stocks should all but eliminate this possibility if your investments are maintained for a minimum five-year period.

This concept is complicated and made even more so by the fact that tax laws are changing constantly (or so it seems). You will *need to consult your own tax adviser before proceeding*. Of course, you must have, or form, a professional corporation to be eligible to take advantage of retained earnings. The decision to incorporate is also a complex one, and many factors besides retained earnings must be considered. But in the decision process that goes into selecting a corporate structure, don't overlook the significant part retained earnings can play in your future financial success.

My retained earnings currently gives my corporation an additional cash flow of over $13,000 annually from dividends alone. Over the years, every stock I have purchased has more than doubled in value (not unusual when investing in stable, high-quality utilities for a good length of time, but certainly not a result you can depend on.) Obviously we didn't obtain all these retained earnings savings our first year of incorporation, but it didn't take many years before we were bumping our heads on the $150,000 retained earnings ceiling. This additional annual revenue provides me with economic freedom, because as sole owner of the corporation I can use the investments and the income they create in any way I choose.

These are tough times financially for many practitioners. I don't know of any one "magic bullet" that will make all the difference for you fiscally. But there are a lot of "little beebees," like retained earnings, that can help. If you are disciplined enough to save and determined enough to figure this out, the result will be more revenue for you and less taxes paid.

Again, the issue is complicated and will require careful study on your part. For those already in a P.C., it is less so. Your main concern is to be *absolutely certain* you never have to pay a penny of corporate tax due to the use of this retained earnings vehicle. *The use of tax losses to offset the income paid out in the form of dividends is critical to this plan's success.*

CHAPTER 21

BONDS—
GOVERNMENT
AND CORPORATE

Owning a stock means you have purchased a portion of the company that sells the stock. You get to vote on some issues that affect the company and are invited, as befits a stockholder-owner, to attend the company's annual meeting. Quarterly and annual reports are sent to you to keep you abreast of your company's performance.

When you purchase a bond, you are simply buying the debt of the issuing entity. In return for your loan, the entity you have "rented" your money to promises to pay you a set amount of interest on predetermined dates in the future. Also at some agreed-upon future date, when the bond has matured or is called, the enterprise will return all of your originally borrowed money to you.

In this chapter we will discuss two types of purchased debt:

1. Government bonds

2. Corporate bonds

A subject near and dear to my investment heart, municipal bonds in all their tax-free glory, will be discussed at length in the following chapter.

Government bonds are simply monies borrowed by our federal government. As sad as it seems, given the state of our nation, these securities are still deemed to be the safest investments in the world. As such, there are no quality ratings for government bonds. They are all backed by the full "faith and trust of the United States Government." (More succinctly they are backed by the government's power to print money and tax, two things of late at which this great nation truly does excel.)

The major distinguishing feature of government bonds is the length of time until a given bond matures. This time period varies from 3 months to 30 years. There are three basic types of government debt. Treasury bills have maturities under one year. Treasury notes mature from 2 to 10 years. Treasury bonds have maturities over 10 years.

You can find government bond listings in your local paper's business section, the *Wall Street Journal,* or my personal favorite publication, *Barron's* (a weekly publication by Dow Jones and Co. that is replete with articles and statistics. I can digest most of the topical financial information I require from this one source in a 60- to 90-minute time investment per week.)

There are also a number of government agencies that have the authority to issue debt in Uncle Sam's name. These include the Federal Farm Credit Bank, Student Loan Market, Federal Home Loan Bank, as well as other smaller agencies listed every week in *Barron's.*

These government agency bonds are also fully supported by our government's taxing muscles. They usually pay a fractionally higher yield than the plain vanilla government bonds, since there is perceived to be a higher risk involved with these issues (one more time: reward = risk). Which agency's paper has the highest yield depends on the public's perception of which arena carries the highest risk at this point in time. Are you curious to know if the risk of nonpayment of debt is perceived to be greater today with students or farmers? Pull out your trusty *Barron's* and note which bond pays the higher yield, and your question will be answered.

I have funded the majority of my retirement plan with government "paper" (bonds). Any money placed in a retirement fund is very illiquid, because there is a penalty established by federal law if these monies are withdrawn prematurely. Generally speaking, you are penalized 10% of any money withdrawn from a retirement plan early. *Early* is usually defined as before age 59½. In addition to the 10% penalty imposed, you would have to pay your regular federal, state, local, social security, Medicare taxes (depressing, isn't it) on the withdrawn assets. Investments you place in any type of retirement plan should be money you are confident you won't need until retirement. The existing tax penalties make it a very expensive resource to withdraw money from.

I want safety at a competitive yield for my retirement funds. Remember, your pension plan is the absolutely last area where you want to take any investment risk. To lose money here reduces the ability of your money, compounding tax free, to grow. I use the government agency bonds to fund my retirement plan if their yields are higher than the more conventional government bonds and notes at the time I wish to invest. The government has guaranteed these agency notes. That promise is where I put my faith, not on the short-term perceptions of possible risk in any given area of our economy involving the different agencies that can temporarily lead to a higher interest yield for that sector.

Years ago, when I was "smarter," I knew if interest rates were going to rise or fall in the near future. I would hold money in the money market funds to invest at the "better yield" (i.e., higher interest rate) which I had ascertained was just about to occur. I'm glad I don't have any idea of how much interest income this "wisdom" cost me. (Remember, the true cost of this lost interest includes the loss of the interest compounding over time, and not just the initial difference of interest lost in, for instance, the first 12-month period.)

Even if I guessed correctly that interest rates were going to rise, I never knew if that increase was going to occur in a month or three years, or how much higher the rates might go. While I waited for the interest "tide" to come in, I usually got a lower rate of interest from my money market fund than I would have received if I had invested longer term right away.

Now when I have cash in my retirement plan, I invest at the best yield I can get the first day I have time to study the possible bond yields available and forget about it. However, if one of you knows the secret to calling the change in interest rates, call me right away *collect*. Such prescience would mean neither of us will ever need to work again. (Please don't feel badly if you can't accurately forecast the direction of interest rates in the future. No one else in the world can either.)

Government bonds can be bought free of any fee or commission directly from the Treasury Department at the time federal auctions are held to sell them. It's a hassle filling out the required government forms. Also, the government sells only new bonds as they are issued, so your selection as to the time frame these bonds will mature over is limited to the maturity dates of the bonds issued at this particular auction.

Brokers or bankers will have available a supply of bonds the government has previously issued for you to pick from, so there will be a wider range of maturities available to make your selection from. You can purchase the bonds on any day you choose and not be forced to wait for the government auction. (Sadly, our government issues debt so often that waiting for a sale doesn't require a lot of patience.)

I always purchase the bonds I want from the bank or broker who is holding my account. The commission they charge for a government bond purchase is small. You simply call your representative and ask them to please buy you the best-yielding government issue with a date of maturity of _____.

That's all it takes. Before I call, I check my newest issue of *Barron's* to compare the yields of the different government bonds available. I tell my broker which of the bonds listed there most appeals to me. He probably won't get that exact bond, but it informs them the length of time to maturity I desire and roughly what yield I'll expect. The yield you will get will be lower than the one quoted in the paper due to the fee you pay your agent to make the purchase. Also, the bonds listed in the paper are being sold in units of millions of dollars. If you need less than a million, as I sometimes do, the yield is slightly lower.

As to how I select the time frame in which I purchase the bonds, I ask your kind indulgence until we get to the concept of *laddering* in the following chapter on municipal bonds.

The advantage of government bonds is their unparalleled safety. They are also in abundant supply due to our government's afore-mentioned insatiable appetite for debt. How competitive the government's yields are compared to other instruments varies with circumstances that affect our economy and thus both interest rates and the investment markets. In times that are perceived as unstable or dangerous, people will pay a premium for safety and desire these government bonds. Remember your old economics about supply and demand? As the demand for these bonds becomes greater, their price increases, and thus the yield they pay declines. Get this critical concept crystal clear in your mind before we proceed. As the price of any bond goes up, the yield they pay decreases.

There is no type of investment you can make that will be as profitable as a retirement plan. There are two main reasons this is so:

1. Our government excuses money placed in retirement funds from all forms of taxation. If you earn $100 and place $10 of that in a *qualified* retirement plan, you only pay tax on $90.

2. The money earned on retirement plan investments compounds tax free.

Some plans, such as IRAs, are very simple and inexpensive to establish. IRAs limit you to a total $4,250 annual contribution for both you and your spouse. IRAs don't involve anyone but you and your spouse; i.e., your office staff is not included in IRA contributions. The main problem with IRAs is that $4,250 annually isn't as significant a contribution toward retirement as many dentists might prefer. Whether $4,250 annually is enough of a contribution for you depends on your retirement goals and how much money you have available to invest. An annual IRA contribution should be the *very minimum* you put aside for retirement. Any bank or broker can set up an IRA plan for you.

Your accountant can tell you about the variety of retirement plans available. Your tax adviser should under no circumstances be selling any financial products, so they are an unbiased source of expert information. Many retirement plan options exist, including 401-k, Keough, and corporate plans to choose among. You will need some professional help in this complex area.

I am in no way trying to suggest a type of retirement plan that is best. "Best" is defined by your personal situation. The critical point I'm trying to make is that creating and funding some type of retirement plan is essential to your financial well-being. Compounding tax-free dollars can't be matched by any other investment return. In addition, the fact that you pay no income tax on money you put into these plans makes them simply unparalleled in their wealth-building ability. Talk to an accountant, and do your homework, but establishing a retirement plan that is right for your situation should be the number one priority investment for almost everyone. I can't stress the advantages of a retirement plan too greatly.

Corporate bonds are debt issued by a corporation, such as General Motors or AT&T. Again, you loan a corporation money, and they agree to pay you a set amount of interest, for a predetermined amount of time, and then return all of your original investment on a predetermined date (the day the bond matures).

There are companies that exist just to rate the quality of bonds. Moody's and Standard and Poor are the best known rating services. The ratings go from AAA, the highest possible rating of quality, to D, the lowest. I never buy any bond with a quality rating below A. If you ever have one bond default (not return your original investment), the extra fractions of a percent yield that you have attained by purchasing the lower quality bonds won't make up for the loss of principal in a lifetime. We'll cover the evaluation of bond quality in great detail in the following chapter on municipal bonds.

Obviously, no corporation is as safe as our government, so due to *higher risk,* corporate bonds should pay a *higher yield.* Again yields will vary with market and economic conditions, as well as the strength of the individual company issuing the bonds. I seldom find a highly rated corporate bond, maturing in the relative short time frame I demand (5 years or less) that offers a big enough yield advantage for me to justify purchasing it instead of a government bond.

As with government securities, these bonds can be purchased from any bank or broker, have low commission prices, and are convenient to buy and hold. If I seem to have paid less than complete attention to investing in corporate bonds, it is because I seldom find them a viable alternative to government bonds in my retirement fund or municipal bonds for my personal investments.

Still, every time I make a purchase of debt (buy a bond) I survey the corporate bonds for possible value. Investment opportunities are perpetually changing. Never make the blunder of thinking that what is true today will be so always.

CHAPTER 22

---◆---

EVERYTHING YOU'VE EVER WANTED TO KNOW ABOUT PURCHASING MUNICIPAL BONDS

It's probably just me, but I'm getting more than a little tired of paying taxes. I don't want to recite the litany of taxes I'm forced to pay; it's just too depressing. Some of them, such as sales tax, our new Medicare tax, or FICA, I can do little about, unless you consider mumbling and grumbling efficacious behavior. But some of those little tax gremlins I can choose *not to pay*. The particular choice I'd like to discuss with you now is the decision you can make to pay no tax *at all*, on income you receive from your personal investments.

Let's be clear as to our objectives here. I purpose to show you a specific technique which will enable you to choose proven, high-quality investments that yield a return *free of all local, state, and federal tax*. When you have digested the information that follows, you should know everything necessary for you personally to purchase these tax-free investments.

We'll begin with a concise review of some generic investment information. My desire is to enable the most neophyte of investors to completely understand our premise. As you recall from Chapter 21, all bonds are *debt*, or said another way, when you buy a bond you loan the entity that issued the bond your money. In contrast, purchasing a stock gives you ownership of a part of the company that issues that specific instrument. Your return on investment when you purchase a stock is tied to the future performance of that company of which you have become a part owner. If the company you have purchased a part ownership in grows, the value of your stock will increase. If the company falls on hard times, the value of its stock can decline. Whatever path the company takes, you and your stock will be along for the ride.

When you purchase a bond, in return for your loan of this money, the borrower agrees to pay you a specific interest rate, at preset intervals, and to return all of your money on the date the bond matures. You may buy bonds from the federal government (no shortage here), from corporations (these cleverly titled Corporate Bonds), or from states, their political subdivisions and certain agencies and authorities: i.e., the aforementioned municipal bonds. The availability of these tax-free municipal bonds allows over 50,000 state and local government units to raise money for needed projects at lower interest rates.

With these facts again fresh in hand, it begs the question, "what's so special about municipal bonds?" The answer is simplicity itself. The interest you receive on "munis" is free from all federal tax, and you pay no state tax if the bond is issued from a government body within the state where you reside. Some cities (New York springs to mind) have local taxes. If you live in New York City and buy a New York City bond, you pay no federal, state, or local taxes on the interest you earn. Get the picture?

There do exist a few *taxable munis*. They have only been issued since the Tax Reform (pardon the oxymoron) Act of 1986 and are a tiny part of the muni spectrum, but you should be aware that they do exist. If you purchase these taxable municipal issues, you'll lose the very tax advantage we are usually looking for. I have bought them for my retirement fund, where no taxes are paid on returns anyway.

Exactly how much does this tax savings amount to? That is the $64,000 question. The answer to this most essential query however, will be different for each of you. To compute your top tax dollar (that is the tax rate you paid on your *most highly* taxed dollar of income), you'll need to review your last federal tax form or cheat and call your accountant and ask him/her what your last year's figures were.

While you lazy people have your accountants on the phone, be sure you also know your state tax rate. This can vary from 0% in a few states that have no state tax up to double digits for a few with high state and local taxes. I live in Illinois. The state tax for Illinois residents is 3%. For me to get an equivalent after-tax yield from a bond issued outside the state of Illinois I must get 1.0211% higher yield.

Personally, I'm not concerned about losing .0211% of yield to state taxes, so I feel free to buy bonds from any state. If I lived in New York City and had to have .093 greater yield from an out-of-state bond to get the same yield as one issued by my city, this would be a much greater concern. State tax is something *you must be aware of,* because it will directly affect your after-tax yield, and maximizing that yield is what this exercise is all about. If you *choose* to purchase bonds from states other than your own, you will pay state taxes on the investment return. In return, you will have a much wider menu of munis to choose from, and this usually means being able to find bonds offering a higher rate of return.

Now that you know your personal federal top tax rate, which is the rate you will pay on all your additional investment income earnings, you'll want to know how taxable and nontaxable yields on the different types of bonds compare on the bottom line, that is, in an after-tax fashion. The table below will let you see in a second how much of a taxable yield you must receive to equal a nontaxed return in your particular tax bracket.

Tax-Free Yield	Taxable Equivalent Yield		
	15%	28%	31% Tax Bracket
4.0%	4.70%	5.55%	5.79%
5.0%	5.88%	6.94%	7.24%
6.0%	7.05%	8.33%	8.69%
7.0%	8.23%	9.72%	10.14%
8.0%	9.41%	11.11%	11.59%
9.0%	10.58%	12.50%	13.04%
10.0%	11.76%	13.88%	14.69%

Let's look at an example. Assume your top dollar is taxed at a 31% rate, and a five-year government bond will yield a 5.80% return. Referring to our table, we see an equivalent tax-free yield would be 4%. In other words, a muni yielding 4% would give you the same after-tax return as a taxable investment yielding a 5.80% return. Remember, this doesn't include state and local tax, which of course can only make the munis' return look better.

A bit of personal philosophy. It is short-sighted to "hate" to pay taxes. This isn't a moral issue, but a financial one. You want to choose the investment course that will give you the *highest after-tax yield possible.* (The redundancy on this point is deliberate.) Buying munis to avoid taxes and ending up with a lower after-tax return is dumb! Stay focused on our goal: the greatest possible after-tax return. For most of you that will mean municipal securities, but each case must be examined in the light of your personal financial situation. My efforts here are directed toward giving you the skills needed to easily make the proper analysis of your own situation, at any point in time.

If you have determined that tax-free yields on munis give you a better true (after-tax) return than it is possible to get with taxable securities, the next logical step is to examine how we purchase these tax-free vehicles. We have two basic choices: invest our money in tax-free municipal bond funds, or purchase the individual bonds themselves.

MUNICIPAL BOND FUNDS

A fund is a group of investments of a similar type purchased in individual units and then placed in one large aggregate pool. Segments of this pool of investments (the fund) are sold to individual investors (us). Professional money managers buy these municipal bonds, in the case of muni funds, and allow you to purchase a tiny part of this large collection of bonds. This gives you *diversity,* so instead of all your dollars being placed in just a few individual bonds (munis sell in units of $5,000), you can own tiny pieces of every bond in the fund. Also, the professional money managers pick the bonds. Because on their prescience, their veritable omniscience, no bond will ever default (fail, or not pay interest) or commit other embarrassing acts in public. The funds are also *convenient.* You don't have to worry about selecting or keeping track of bonds, and it `s possible to start investing in a fund for as little as $500.

"Conventional Wisdom" (I must confess, she and I are merely passing acquaintances) has it that if you have less than $25,000 to invest, a fund is the place for you to begin. Surely, this is the case if you have less than $5,000 to invest, because this is the least amount of capital you can purchase an individual bond with.

My duty done to Ms. Conventional, let me acknowledge that I am not a supporter of bond funds. For this reason (and probably for a lot of other reasons I'd rather not reflect on), I don't feel competent to recommend a specific fund to you. These funds are advertised in places like *Barron's*, the *Wall Street Journal*, or any of the plethora of business magazines such as *Forbes* or *Money Magazine*, so it isn't hard to obtain information about them.

I could expound at length about my reasons for not investing in muni funds. For example, these funds, even the no-loads (no-load means no sales charge is billed to you when you purchase shares of the funds), charge a significant management fee which reduces the yield you get from your investment. But for the sake of brevity, let me limit my discussion to one major problem with using funds, as I perceive it. In effect, purchasing a bond fund is hiring someone else (an expert, of course), to do your thinking for you.

Now let me hasten to add, I deplore thinking as much as any of you! But let's be optimists and assume that you some day will have a significant amount of money in municipal bonds. When will you learn to purchase them yourself? If you abdicate your responsibility to others, be it spouse, staff, lawyer, or investment professional, you limit your personal growth. My question to you: *do you really want your financial future controlled by others?* That choice may place you on a road slippery with the tears of many fellow travelers.

I guess if you never plan to have any money anyway, the point is moot. However, if by any chance you think you may some day have a positive net worth, I'd encourage you to begin to study the following steps and obtain the knowledge necessary to purchase the individual bonds themselves.

INDIVIDUAL MUNICIPAL BONDS

WARNING: to complete this section you will have to study (just a little, right here), gather some information, and *reach a conclusion!* It is possible you could make a mistake! It's also conceivable that you'll do a few simple things right and learn in the process. That caveat stated, I can however promise you this information is a lot easier and much more interesting than figuring out OSHA regulations.

Quality is our first concern. Young investors may wish this tattooed to their forehead! Allow me to touch again on a critical point. Remember the best advice any investor ever accepted: it's not the rate of return that is critical, but the *return of principal.* In other words, the main objective is to get your money back!

How can we accurately, quickly, and consistently judge this, by far the most critical of concerns with any investment, quality? Here is a very pleasant surprise: we don't have to for munis (or for the corporate bonds we've just discussed), because the same rating system done by the same people applies to them also. There exist agencies that do this task for us and do a much better job than any individual could possibly do.

Standard and Poor is the rating agency most often quoted by the individuals selling bonds, and I personally buy only bonds rated A or better by this venerable company. *With this single bit of information you have solved over 90% of the quality issue.*

There remain two items to consider regarding the quality of your investment. There are two basic types of munis:

1. *Government Obligations, or GOs.* These are backed by both borrowing and taxing power. Whoever issues these bonds has the ability and desire to tax people to make them meet the bond's obligations. You don't have to be very concerned about quality with GOs. I believe we all understand how taxes work well enough to appreciate that fact.

2. *Revenue Bonds.* These plan to pay the interest and principal back to bondholder based on money (revenue) raised from whatever project your bond "loan" helped to build. These can be fine, especially if they are for "essential services" such as water or sewer works. There is little chance of people choosing to do without either. I avoid hospital and nursing-home bonds, unless of the highest quality rating. For whatever reasons, health care issues have had the highest rate of muni defaults.

One final issue as pertains to municipal bond quality: some bonds are protected by their own insurance. The bond issuer pays about .15%

(The bond yield is reduced this much. If your bond would have paid 5% yield, it now returns 4.85%.) to achieve this added protection. The insurance is to guarantee the interest and principle will be repaid, even if the project itself fails to meet its fiduciary responsibilities.

With the support of insurance, the quality rating of these bonds will invariably be AAA (the highest rating). But why is this insurance needed? How good are the insurance companies' guarantee and financial strength? How many other bonds have they guaranteed, and what happens if several fail? (Remember, top quality bonds don't spend their money on this insurance.) I don't know the answers to these questions, and thus I tend to not buy insured bonds.

Some bonds are not rated for quality. These are marked N.R. (Not Rated). Brokers may assure you these bonds are safe. I tell the broker he can purchase them; I'm not interested. Nothing is more important with bonds than high quality, which guarantees the return of our investment.

Now that we can safely pick the quality of bonds we're comfortable with, the next question we must answer is how many years do we want the bond to extend out in time before the bond matures and we get our original investment back? There is no right or wrong answer to this query, but I will share with you some general guidelines and my personal philosophy.

Money that I place in any type of bond I completely expect to stay invested in those bonds until they mature and the money is returned to me. I don't want to ever have to sell these bonds before maturity. This is critical! Munis are *no place* for money you're not absolutely sure you won't need in the short term. You can sell munis at any time, but if forced to do so, you take two risks:

1. The market for munis is not a "level playing field." If you call three brokers and ask them what your specific bond is worth at that moment in time (and if you ever do have to sell a bond, call at least three sources and get competitive bids), I promise you'll get three different figures. (Sell to the highest, right?) This uncertainty as to what constitutes a fair price is best avoided by never needing to sell a bond.

2. As with *any kind of bond*, their value for resale will vary with the overall interest rates. If you buy a bond at a time when a fair rate of return is 5%, and when you wish to sell that bond,

the going rate of interest for a similar bond is 6%, then the price of the bond you own (with the 5% coupon), will decrease until its yield reaches the current 6% rate. If you paid $1,000 for your bond, its value would decrease by one-sixth in our example to approximately $830 in current value.

Remember, *no one knows* when interest rates will move or in what direction. If people tell you they know the future direction interest rates will take, rest assured, *they'll lie to you about other things too.*

The point here: invest in all bonds only with money you won't need to use in the near future. There are people who buy bonds expressly to "play" these interest rates, and if they guess correctly the direction of the next interest rate move, they can make fortunes. These individuals are speculators. We are *savers.* You can sell bonds if you must, but you could lose part of your principal! Loss of principal is an investment event to be avoided at all costs!

Remember your lessons from Chapter 18. If you want the advantage of munis' tax-free status, along with complete liquidity, put your money in municipal money market funds. Usually the rates for these funds will be much lower than in longer term bonds, but you will be certain to get all of your invested dollars back whenever you choose.

But our subject was *time.* How long a time to maturity should my bond carry? Usually, the longer out the time continuum you go, the greater the interest return you will get. (Allow me to skip over inverted yield curves. I can't recall one since Mr. Carter ran things.) Basically, the greater return for a longer period of time to maturity is to compensate for increased risk. The longer an investment is held, the more likely it is that something could occur to reduce the value of your investment.

I personally tend to buy bonds with around a five-year length of maturity (a March 1993 purchase would be mature in March 1998).

This is just my personal preference and has no basis in absolute wisdom. I modify this time frame based on my perception (read guess) of prevailing interest rates. If rates are historically low, as they have been in 1992 and 1993, I buy shorter maturities, often around three years. I hope in three years that interest rates will have increased, and when my current bond matures I can reinvest at a higher rate of return.

When rates are historically high, I *may* go out to seven or eight years to maturity, to "lock in" those higher returns. Remember, anyone who tells you which way rates will move in the future will lie to you about other things too.

A concept that helps eliminate the risk of all your bonds coming due (maturing) at the same time, i.e., at the lowest moment in the history of bond yields, is called *laddering*. This simply means that you stagger or ladder the maturity rates of bonds to balance out their times to maturity. If you have $50,000 in bonds and want to go out a maximum of 5 years in maturity, you will have $10,000 invested in each year. As the oldest bond matures, you reinvest this capital at the far end of your bond portfolio time "ladder."

Some bonds are sold with *calls*. This simply means the company that issued the bond has the right to repay your money early on a prearranged date, if it chooses to do so. Well, you get all your money back when a bond is called. Sounds harmless? Not at all. If interest rates have gone up, they won't exercise the call, because to borrow money would be more expensive for the bond issuer now than to continue to pay the current rate of interest on the bond you previously purchased. They will only exercise the call if interest rates have dropped. Now they can borrow at cheaper rates. When you reinvest the capital they return by redeeming your bond at the earlier call date, you will receive less interest in return.

In short, calls can potentially be of help to the company issuing the bond, but to the owner of the bond, they can do nothing but hurt. There is *no* upside potential for you. I'm married and have four kids. I don't need any more deals like that. *No calls allowed.* (Some bonds can be called, but only at a price higher than the bond was originally issued for. You may have bought the bond for $5,000, and at some point before the maturity date, the issuer can refund your money at, say, 102% of the purchase price. Most calls are at the face value of the bond, so be certain if there is a call option, that you will get this premium price. The total return on a bond subject to a call is referred to as yield-to-call return. You must know the yield-to-call return if you purchase a callable bond, because this is the actual return you receive should the company exercise their call option.)

Yield-to-maturity is the overall investment return on a bond held to maturity. You can purchase a bond for more than its face value (over $5,000). Such a bond is said to be purchased at a *premium*, and your yield-to-maturity is thus reduced. (You buy a bond at $5,200. When it matures you get $5,000, or the face value of the bond back.) Some bonds are sold at a *discount*, or less than the $5,000 face value. Buying a bond at a discount increases your yield-to-maturity. (Let's say your purchase price was $4,800. When the bond matures you receive the face value of $5,000. Your $200 gain is taxable.) Be sure when you receive a quote on the bond yield that you know not only the interest rate paid, but the yield-to-maturity if the bond is not selling at par. (Par is the original price of issue and the amount of the money paid out when the bond is redeemed, regardless of the purchase price. Par is always $5,000 for munis.)

How much will it cost you in commissions to buy your $5,000 bond? Good question, but one difficult to answer. Let me quote from a chart published in the *Wall Street Journal*. These are their numbers for the commission a financial adviser earns on a $10,000 investment.

Municipal, Corporate, or Government Bond: $50–$100
Common Stock on NYSE: $200–$250
Annuities, Life Insurance policies: $400–$600
Limited Partnerships: $600–$1000

There are a lot more variations than this possible when purchasing any security, but this chart serves us as a rough guide. Maybe the best answer to, How much do I pay to purchase a bond? is, Usually not as much as for other investments.

It may be a coincidence, but you'll find some brokers and their ilk will want to sell you about anything but a low commission muni. They will have all kinds of more daring investments to offer that a person of your obvious wit and wisdom can appreciate. I reiterate: It is completely fair to ask what their commission is on this intriguing concept they are advancing for your consideration. Do patients hesitate to ask what your fees are? The sales person probably will hem and haw and never tell you anyway, but it's a good way to get back to discussing bonds.

This segues nicely to our last point: *Where and how do I purchase these bonds?*

Where is easy. Any brokerage house, such as Merrill Lynch, Dean Witter, or Piper Jaffray or almost any bank or savings and loan will sell bonds to you.

The muni market differs from equities, where the price you pay for a share of a given major stock will be the same at a given time no matter whom you purchase it from. (Remember, if you buy 100 shares of AT&T at 9 A.M. on Tuesday, you will pay the same price, except for commission, no matter where or from whom you make your purchase.) With munis, dealers may sell only what they have themselves purchased or at least have available to purchase. Also, you won't see a commission fee charge on your transaction slip as you will with a stock purchase. That fee is taken out of the price of the bond, so you never really know what commission you have paid. For top quality bonds, the commission will range from .25% to 1%. For poor quality, or junk bonds, on which the greedy and foolish will *risk their principal*, you could be charged up to 3% for the dubious privilege of this purchase.

Because of these vagaries, you must always contact at least three sources (brokers, bankers, or S & Ls) and get a bid from each.

Let's make the selection and purchase of a municipal bond so simple that any child (and thus, we hope, a dentist) could do it.

1. You know your own personal tax rate, both state and federal. You cheated and asked your accountant, even though the information is clearly stated on your tax return. That's why you pay accountants, right?

2. You have consulted the accompanying table that compares tax-exempt and taxable yields. You can look in *any* newspaper and see what a government bond yield is (in the business section of all but the smallest papers), or call the local bank and ask what CDs or government bonds are yielding for your desired length of time to maturity. Remember, we buy tax free *only if our after-tax yield is superior.*

3. You have a time frame you feel comfortable with and are as sure as humanly possible you won't have to cash the bond before it reaches maturity and risk some of your principal.

4. You have picked out a *minimum* of three potential sources to buy bonds from.

Here's how your phone call will go, word for word.
"Hello, Mr. Smith. My name is Dr.———." (They like the "Doctor"

part. It usually means the caller has money and doesn't know how to handle it. This guy will find out differently in about one minute. You're now a pro!)

"I'd like a price quote from you on the purchase of $—— (remember, munis come in $5,000 units) of municipal bonds. I want to consider only A or better quality, and I want the bonds to mature on or about —— —— (your selected date). Please advise me if the bond you recommend is insured. *I want you to be aware that I am opening this investment to three competitive bids.* Please call me back at this number when you have complete information about your possible selections."

Informing the dealer that you are accepting competitive bids means you'll get their best price. They live on commissions from sales, and no sale = no commission. The broker may want to keep you on the phone as he reviews his bond list. I want them to take their time and give me their best information, so I insist they return my call.

After a while you'll eliminate some potential sources of munis because the individuals employed there don't want to work with you. Often these are people who don't answer your specific questions, but instead try to sell you something other than what you called about. There are thousands of people who sell munis. Don't hesitate to sever a relationship you're not comfortable in.

With time you'll also find true professionals that are a pleasure to work with. However, never fail to get at least three competitive bids, and inform the broker you are doing so. You can like a broker personally, but this is business. Losing the sale to a better deal is healthy to the broker-buyer relationship. It keeps them on their toes.

One last point: the future of munis. I'll ask you for a quick gaze into your crystal ball. Do you expect taxes to go up or down in the near future? If you suspect up (you clever devil, you), such a change would make munis more valuable. (If you suspect taxes will be going down in the near future, I'm with you in spirit, and I hope medication will help your condition.)

CHAPTER 23

THE VERY BEST WAY TO PAY FOR YOUR CHILD'S EDUCATION USING THE UNIFORMED GIFT TO MINORS ACT (UGMA)

Do you ever stop and ask yourself: *why do you do it?* Why subject yourself to the daily grind (which often leaves me at the point of near exhaustion) that is modern dentistry? Certainly there is no simplistic answer to so complex a question, but I would be willing to bet that most of you parents reading this are just like me. All of the work, worry, and frustration that makes up our career is worth it, if by doing so we can provide the things we value for our loved ones.

One of the most, if not the singularly most important benefit we can provide for our children, is help in acquiring a fine education. I am proud to say that I worked my way through eight years of college, paying all of my own expenses. I'm sure of two things:

1. The experience strengthened me. (Nietzsche said, "that which does not kill instructs." I'm not dead, so I must have learned from the journey.)

2. I don't want anyone I love to ever have to go through anything like that.

It follows then, that Mom and I will be paying at least part of what is becoming an increasingly larger bill for education. Our situation is a worse case scenario. We have four kids, all pretty smart. I'm afraid just four years won't be enough college for any of them.

Let's see if we are in agreement so far:

1. We love our children and want the best for them.

2. What is "best" must include an excellent education.

3. We are probably going to be required to pay for at least a major portion of that investment.

If we agree on these premises, let's attack the conundrum of finding the best possible way to pay for Junior's college years. I believe we can solve this dilemma using the how-to-eat-an-elephant technique of problem-solving; i.e., one bite at a time.

BITE 1. How much will this investment in education cost? The answer to this query requires either guess work or prescience. T. Roe Price Associates, evidently skilled in at least one of the two afore-named disciplines, has developed the following table to help us in this regard. I hope it won't scare you to death. The company assumed a 7% annual inflation of college expenses in its "guesstimation." Let's all hope and pray that it estimate is high, if not downright extreme, but it would be better to be over-, rather than underfunded, when it comes time to make this significant investment in our children's future.

Table 23–1.
How much to save for your child's college

Years until college	4-year total cost		Monthly savings	
	Public	**Private**	**Public**	**Private**
1	$ 38,343	$ 80,891	$3,059	$6,454
2	$ 41,027	$ 86,553	$1,527	$3,315
3	$ 43,899	$ 92,612	$1,076	$2,270
4	$ 46,972	$ 99,095	$ 828	$1,747
5	$ 50,260	$106,031	$ 679	$1,434
6	$ 53,778	$113,454	$ 581	$1,225
7	$ 57,543	$121,395	$ 510	$1,076

Years until college	4-year total cost		Monthly savings	
	Public	**Private**	**Public**	**Private**
8	$ 61,571	$129,893	$ 457	$ 964
9	$ 65,881	$138,986	$ 416	$ 877
10	$ 70,492	$148,714	$ 383	$ 808
11	$ 75,427	$159,125	$ 356	$ 751
12	$ 80,707	$170,263	$ 333	$ 703
13	$ 86,356	$182,182	$ 314	$ 663
14	$ 92,401	$194,943	$ 298	$ 629
15	$ 98,869	$208,580	$ 284	$ 599
16	$105,790	$223,180	$ 271	$ 573
17	$113,195	$238,803	$ 260	$ 549
18	$121,119	$255,519	$ 251	$ 529
19	$129,597	$273,406	$ 242	$ 510
20	$138,669	$292,544	$ 234	$ 493

1. Costs based on the College Board's Annual Survey of Colleges for the 1992–93 school year and include tuition, room and board, transportation, books and other expenses. In-state residence is assumed for public schools.

2. Tables assume 7% annual increase in college costs and an 8% after-tax annual return on investment (8.3% based on monthly compounding). No additional investments are assumed once the child starts school, and investments are made at the beginning of each year.

As you can see, if your darling is off to school next year, you will need about $38,000 to pay for four years in a public, or state-run, institution. If your child is more discerning, you will be required to fork over roughly $81,000 for the privilege of four years at a private school. This *assumes* your child will be finished with all of his or her higher education expenses in four years.

But let's say you're proud parents of a newborn, potential genius. Just looking into her eyes you can already tell she is smart, if not downright gifted! What will the ticket be for her 18 years from now? Again resorting to our table, we see a paltry $121,119 if she goes the plebeian, public route or (God forbid) $255,519 for a private school. (At least at these prices, it should keep out the riff raff!)

That's bite one. Take a moment to quit shaking. No, it's not legal to sell your children. Maybe they'll be dumb or run away from home.

Maybe you want to mentally review your position on birth control. As soon as you've eliminated all those distractions, let's return to our elephant. As you can see, we've got work to do.

BITE 2. The best way to pay for your child's education. Let me now define that pesky term, *best*. I mean simply the cheapest possible way to pay for your child's education figured in *after-tax dollar cost* to you. I'm afraid I have no ability to make the schools cheaper, but I can make some suggestions to help you pay their egregious bills for the smallest possible real cost.

Let's start by looking at the "worst" way to pay. Your kids are already in college, and you have no savings. You pay their bills as best you can using *after-tax dollars*. Let's examine this scenario more closely.

You perform $100 of fine dental care. Because you're a nice guy (and perhaps overpay your staff), overhead is 65%, so you have $35 remaining after the office bills are paid. You still have FICA, Medicare, state, and federal taxes to pay, so let's estimate you will have $18 remaining after fulfilling your legal obligations. Because you have kids in college, your family no longer eats or has a home, so the entire $18 goes to the college fund. Such a plan, of earning and paying as the child goes through school, calls for a great sacrifice in lifestyle, and costs the most money. *Worst* is easy to define.

With best you begin to save when your child is very small, preferably at birth. (Maybe after reviewing our table you might begin saving at conception.) You and your wife can both *gift* $10,000 apiece to every one of your children each year, tax free. (That's $20,000 per year for the two of you gifted tax free annually to each child, but if you can afford to do that you sure don't need to finish this little story!)

The amount you'll need to finally have available for Junior you can estimate from the accompanying table. Two things are critical to our savings plan:

1. We must begin to save early, to take advantage of compounding interest.

2. To use the least possible dollars (and thus deserve the coveted "best" title), the money must be allowed to build up tax free.

Let's look at compounding first. To get a fairly accurate idea of how your money will grow we'll use the Rule of 72. Do you recall how this handy little mathematical shortcut allows you to figure how quickly your invested money will double (or your debt will double if you choose to look at such depressing things) by dividing the percent of interest you are earning (or paying) into the number 72? (Don't ask me why this works, I'm a dentist. But if you take out your calculator and test it a few times, you'll be surprised at its accuracy.)

An example, please. Junior has just been born, but that's long enough for you to certify him/her as a budding genius, fall completely in love and want only the absolute best for this budding protégé. (Of course, veteran parents know all of this will change dramatically by the teen years, but that issue isn't really germane to our point.) College will be here in 18 short years. How much do we need to save now for that great future day? It all depends on the interest your investment can earn.

Let's say you invest in a financial instrument that pays a 10% return. Ten divided into 72 = 7.2. Your money doubles every 7.2 years. In 18 years every thousand dollars you put away will be worth roughly $6,000. (At 7.2 years; $1,000 becomes $2,000. By 14.4 years this has doubled again to $4,000. In the remaining 3.6 years we can estimate a 50% increase to $6,000.)

What if you took the $1,000 and bought a hot stock? What if over the eighteen years it grew at a 24% rate? Divide 72 by 24 and you get 3 years. Your money doubles every three years for 18 years! Your $1,000 has become $64,000!

Take a break and play with the numbers a little bit yourself, but get an idea of the *power of compounding interest.*

But wait a minute. By what legerdemain did we shake off the debilitating effects of the pesky tax man? Pay close attention here. We gifted the money to Junior using something called the Uniformed Gift to Minors or Uniform Transfer to Minors Act, hereafter to be referred to as UGMA.

You *have to have professional help here.* The regulations on how these plans are set up differ from state to state. UGMAs are simple to do, however, and there is usually no fee involved. Specific property (this could be cash, bonds, stocks, etc.) is deeded over to the child in an *irrevocable trust.* Once this simple form is completed the property belongs to the child, and all the income it produces is taxed to them.

But what is the child's tax rate? Here the wicket gets sticky. Tax laws were enacted in 1986 that have reduced the benefits of these plans and made the tax picture more difficult to deal with (another "tax simplification effort" by our great solons in public office!). In analyzing the tax situation, we have to make two distinctions: Is the child over or under 14 years of age (should be fairly easy for a parent), and is the income earned or unearned?

Unearned income is what we're dealing with here. It's interest, dividends, etc.; all similar in the fact that they aren't wages. For children under the age of 14, a certain amount of this unearned income is subject to a Standard Deduction. The amount of this deduction has been raised every year. In 1990 it was $500, in 1991 it was raised to $550. The 1992 total is $600. You could venture a guess as to the 1993 deduction, as there does seem a trend, but as of this writing, the actual figure for 1993 has not been set.

This standard deduction means that if your child had unearned income below $600 in 1992, no taxes are to be paid, and no tax return needs to be filed. If unearned income is $601 or more, a return must be filed. If in the calendar year your child's *total income*, both earned and unearned, exceeds $600, a return must be filed, even if the unearned portion was $1. The exact taxes paid on income over this $601 figure get very complex, but they are paid at the *parents' tax rate*, which for the income above $600, acts to dilute the tax advantages we are so desperately seeking.

Once your children are over 14 years of age, they still keep the $600 standard deduction on unearned income and can earn in wages or salary up to $3,600 tax free. Also, now anything over $601 is taxed at their tax rate of 15%, not at the parent's higher level.

Establishing the UGMA trust itself, as I mentioned, is simple and usually free of any fees or charges. But, it is *irrevocable*. Once the assets are given, they can't be taken back. There is also a risk that the laws will once again be changed to punish the innocent. ("We're from the government, and we're here to help.") You will also need tax advice from your accountant as to how to proceed with your plan. All these negatives being accounted for, go back and reread the worst case again. Review the chart estimating college costs. For the majority of us, this is still the best possible option available to help fund our children's educational needs.

BITE 3. What do we invest in to get the best possible return for our children? Almost any property will qualify. Books could be written on all the possibilities, but let's look at a few excellent choices. These are all financial instruments I have used or am currently using in my own kids' plans.

ZERO COUPON BONDS (ZEROS)

I guess the original zeros were U.S. Savings Bonds. You buy zeros for a portion of their face value. [I.e., you pay $50 for a bond that is worth $100 when it matures. The length of time to maturity will vary by the rate of interest being paid as our Rule of 72 has illustrated. The annual interest being "paid" on zeros isn't actually received by you, but instead increases the value of the bonds. If you invested in a bond paying 10% interest, in the first year your $50 bond becomes worth $55, and while you receive no money (unless you cash the bond in), you must pay taxes on this $5 of earnings. This makes the zeros a *terrible* investment in an account, such as your personal savings, that is taxable. You have to pay taxes on money you haven't even gotten yet! It makes a lot of sense in college funds or retirement plans of any type, where taxes on your investment returns are deferred.]

The advantage of zero is that the interest is automatically reinvested at the coupon rate of the bond. Instead of getting a $5 check from your bond and having to find something to invest that minuscule amount of cash in, the interest stays in the bond and earns the same rate of return as your initial $50 purchase did until the bond is cashed or matures.

Because both the face value and the return rate is guaranteed, you can tell precisely to the day and dollar how much this bond will be worth when you need it, on that great day when Junior heads for school. You will know that the bond will be worth exactly the face amount of the bond on the agreed-upon day of maturity you established when you initially purchased your investment. This makes financial planning a lot more simple.

You can buy zeros from any broker, S & L, or bank. Usually the bonds you purchase are U.S. Government securities, still considered to be the safest investment in the world.

SERIES EE BONDS

These government savings bonds are a form of zeros too, but with a special twist. They have some unique features designed specifically for college savings plans.

These bonds can also be bought from any bank or S & L, but not from stock brokers. One nice feature: there is no fee or cost to buy or sell these bonds. Another positive feature is that the bonds pay a guaranteed minimum interest rate that increases the longer you hold the bond. If you cash the bond less than six months from the date of purchase, you will receive no interest. You must be absolutely certain that you won't need any funds you invest in these bonds until at least six months from the date you purchased them.

As of March 1st, 1993 EE bonds pay a minimum yield of 4%. The return you get can increase, based on the return of what the government refers to as a "market basket average." This is a composite of yields tied to the rates being paid on intermediate U.S. Treasury bonds. So while the 4% is a guaranteed minimum you can receive, if rates on intermediate government securities increase while you're holding the EE bonds, your return will automatically be increased.

Two warnings:

1. The government can change these minimum amounts on *new bonds* being issued if it chooses to. It can't change the return on bonds that have already been sold.

2. Interest is paid *only* twice a year on these bonds, unlike some investments that compound interest returns on a daily basis. If you cash in the bond a day before the scheduled payment date, you will get no interest for the last six months you've held the bonds.

The federal tax situation with EE bonds is where the neat twist occurs. If you use the proceeds from the bond for college expenses within the year the bond is cashed, you pay no federal tax on the bond's earnings. This money is completely tax free to single tax payers with adjusted gross incomes under $44,150, and then the percent of tax-free return begins to decline until at $59,150 none of the interest is tax free. For married and joint filing accounts, interest is tax free up to $66,200 and tapers off until none is tax free at a $99,200 level of AGI.

While it is true that many of us are fortunate enough to have incomes that limit or eliminate this tax break, it is there for those with lower adjusted gross incomes who need it most. Even without the federal-tax savings, the rate of return being paid now for a safe investment with a guaranteed minimum return and the possibility of increase makes it an attractive option. Also, the interest is always state and local tax free.

You can find your adjusted gross income on your federal tax return, and you get more information on EE Bonds by calling 1-800-4US-BOND. Any local bank or S & L will also be glad to give you this information. Buying EEs simply means filling out a short form at the bank or S & L. You are limited to purchasing $15,000 in actual dollar cost per year (this is $30,000 face or maturity value of the bond).

Bonds are safe and sure, if somewhat boring investments. The last idea I want to share with you is more complex and difficult, but can reward you with a potentially much greater return.

STOCKS

As we've discussed, when you purchase a stock, you are buying a part of the company. If the company prospers and grows, the value of the stock increases. Some, but not all, stocks pay a dividend. This is a certain dollar amount paid to each holder of a share of stock, usually on a quarterly basis. Stock dividends can be raised in good times, but also lowered or eliminated in bad times. Thus a stock dividend's rate of return is not guaranteed, as are bond payments.

As we've discussed, stock returns, especially over longer periods of time, have out-performed the returns on bonds. Unfortunately what is true for an average isn't necessarily true for any particular stock during any given time frame. Stocks, due to the potential growth in a company, can offer you larger rewards than bond investments, but selecting them is much more of an art, and there is always a risk that the price of the stock could decline.

If you consider funding your precious college fund with stocks, pick ones of the highest quality. There are many high-quality stocks that have increased in value over the years, while paying a dividend of 5% or more. Once again, stocks can be bought from brokers (like Dean Witter or Merrill Lynch) or from most banks and S & Ls today. No, I can't tell you which stocks to buy. I can repeat Will Rogers' sage advice: buy stocks that are going up in price, and sell them for more than you paid. If they aren't going up, don't buy them!

PERSONALLY SPEAKING

I will share with you what I have done with my own four kids' money. I have used all three of these instruments (stocks, zeros, and EE bonds) at varied times. My younger kids' funds all started when they were born with AT&T stock. I bought it when the "Baby Bells" first split off from the parent company. I paid $17 a share for the stock, and at the time of this writing, it's worth $60-plus per share. Many stocks have done better, but my kids and I are happy with this return.

I put money in zeros at the same time I purchased a part of Ma Bell. It was hard to bite the bullet and put money away when my kids were infants. A vacation or new car would have been nice. Now that two of the kids are in college, I'm glad I made the decision to put a few thousand dollars away at the time. Certainly the investment (believe me, it felt like a sacrifice at the time) has paid great dividends.

Using a *combination* of stock (with a greater potential return, yet greater risks) and zeros (safer and more predictable, yet no hedge against the kind of inflation we lived in during the Carter years) seemed to me a sensible approach. As my older kids got closer to college age, I cashed in the stocks and placed the money in EE bonds. I don't get the federal tax savings due to my tax level, but the zeros are convenient to work with, and the return is completely predictable. Since you can buy them in a series of bonds at face amounts as low as $100, I can cash in whatever amount of the bonds I need for school costs at the moment, and not disturb the rest of the investment. This combination of flexibility and liquidity is helpful.

Let me dare to end this chapter with a little personal philosophy. Note it is labeled as such. When my two oldest started college, they clearly understood that they had a certain amount of dollars available to them in their college funds. They also understood that this was all the support they would get from us financially. They were free to spend it as they chose. If they went to state schools, the money would go farther. If they graduated quickly, more would be left for them to use for other things (such as graduate schools).

I like this approach because I didn't have to keep saying yes or no. Yes, you can go to Harvard, or no, you can't. I have never even asked them for an accounting of how the money was spent.

Maybe you've heard that kids can't get through school in four years anymore. Too tough. Can't be done. Well, my kids "can't" finish college in four years either. John, Jr. graduated in 3½ years with honors and has been accepted into law school. Heather is on course to graduate in three years, and has a 3.91 GPA on a four-point scale.

Did our decision on the way we chose to finance their school expenses improve their college performance? I don't know. I do know that my children became responsible for their own finances, and they handled it very well. And, after all, what greater learning experience can any educational system provide than to teach the lesson that you are responsible for your own life?

I wish the matters we've just discussed weren't so complex, but investing and taxes are two subjects that don't lend themselves to simplicity. You will need help from accountants, bankers, or brokers. These are decisions both important and difficult to make. I wish you the best.

CHAPTER 24

FINANCIAL LOSSES
I HAVE KNOWN

(And a Few I've Only Read About)

I can think of things I'd rather do than relive for your benefit the financial ventures I have lost money on over the years. I'm committing this unnatural act, because in conversations with dentists across these fruited plains, I have repeatedly heard horror stories of investment misadventures they have lived through. It seems most of us have experienced financial setbacks, but few wish to admit it. Instead these misadventures are left out of the cocktail prattle, which usually features us as financial geniuses.

However, it is only by being aware of the potential dangers that exist in the investment arena that we can hope to avoid such difficulties ourselves. Remember the story about the Indian boy and the rattlesnake? Well, if you decide to pick up an investment snake (and many of you will), I want to be sure you can at least identify these rattlers when you see them. Then you won't be an innocent victim, only a stupid one.

I'm sad to say that it is somewhat difficult for me to know where to begin the story of my investment setbacks. I've had my share of financial fiascos. My original investment decision, in those halcyon days when I first realized I actually had some money left over to invest after all my bills were paid, was to diversify. My theory was that by each year studying new types of investments I would learn about them all. I did. I learned there are many ways to lose money in this world.

My initial selection among the potential fields for investment was chosen by my accountant. He informed me that I had a "tax problem." I later came to realize that this is accountant-speak for "You are making money and paying taxes." *This is a key point. Most accountants perceive making money and paying taxes to be a troublesome thing.* As my experiences recounted in this chapter will so ably illustrate, you can be afflicted with worse problems than paying taxes. One I can think of off the top of my head is having no money.

Employing an excellent accountant is a must for any chance of financial success in the world of modern dentistry. Today's tax codes are beyond my comprehension, and professional help in dealing with tax matters is essential. Accountants may also find the answers to complex financial questions for you. No business deal can be considered without an understanding of the tax ramifications inherent in the venture.

However, accountants are not trained in investing! Follow their advice and you deserve what you'll get: lots of tax losses. Accountants are asked by doctors who are less informed about financial matters than the CPAs for advice on investing. Accountants seem to feel they should attempt to accommodate these requests. This is where the ball of yarn begins to unravel. If you look to accountants, lawyers, or financial planners to do your investment thinking for you, it will cost you dearly. Take advice and help from them, but *you have to think and reach the final investment decisions by yourself.*

So accountants are critical to your success. Also critical is the fact that you must understand and follow up on the advice they give you personally. Last year, when I reviewed my taxes before mailing them in, I found no mistakes made by my accountant in their preparation. This is the *first time* that has ever happened! Every year but this one, we have had to redo my taxes before they were sent in due to errors in their preparation I unearthed while reviewing the completed forms. It takes me a couple of hours to look my tax returns over *after* they are filled out. I don't enjoy reviewing them, but every year I do. I have never been audited. I believe the connection between my extra care on tax returns and the IRS's lack of interest in my finances to be more than coincidence.

I've avoided the topic of my financial losses as long as I can. Did you get my point? *You* make the investment mistakes, not your paid minions. Now, bravely on to tax loss number one.

OIL AND GAS LIMITED PARTNERSHIPS

Oil and gas drilling programs were my first investments. The selection of gas and oil alone violated *every* rule of investing I have tried to teach you. I was seeking a tax shelter to avoid the terrible problem my accountant had pointed out to me, that most egregious of sins, making money and paying taxes. *Never invest to avoid taxes. The only reason for anyone to invest is to make a profit.* If your profit-making investment also yields a tax break, so much the better. But committing money *just* to reduce taxes and losing on the investment will end up reducing your net worth. That point seems so simple and obvious that I really can't explain why it is constantly being ignored, especially by doctors.

As I began my investment career, I looked over each prospectus from oil and gas companies as if I was studying for a final examination. I painstakingly reviewed the information from six companies. I did my best to pick the best two companies to invest in. With the hours I devoted to the task, I probably did select the best two investment choices. This fact simply illustrates that more than likely the companies were all bad investments. It is very hard to feel joyful over selecting the best among a group of poor investments.

Oil and gas limited partnerships are programs designed to explore for oil and gas. The limited partner (that's you) puts up the money that allows the drilling to take place. You have no control over what the company does; hence the term limited. As a limited partner you are also protected from any debt the company may incur, but not be able to pay. The debtor has no recourse to you, but only to the oil and gas company itself. That key phrase means no one has the right to extract from you money beyond your initial investment. That's part of the good news, that all you can lose within the limited partnerships' agreement is your entire investment!

Limited partnerships are usually "highly speculative" investments. Says so right in the prospectus. You have to fill out a form stating you have a certain net worth and/or a certain annual income to have the privilege of risking your money on these ventures. Sadly, they don't require an I.Q. test to see if you qualify to invest. The biggest risk is that of not finding any oil when they drill wells. This risk is reduced as these programs drill a lot of wells; 50 would be a good average. If just a few of these 50 wells hit a lot of oil, you could have a very pleasant financial outcome.

The reward, other than the obvious chance to make income if oil is discovered, is that you get an immediate tax deduction in the year you make the investment. Also, part of the income you earn if oil is found is tax free, due to something called the depletion allowance (you don't really want to know all that much about these things).

I invested in two programs. This deliberate decision to diversify showed excellent instincts for a neophyte investor. One program did well, and after about 10 years passed, I made money. Not as much as I could have made had I purchased a bond and let the money compound for me. I have had no realistic way to get the money out of the program if I wished to (totally un-liquid, right?). But eventually I did make money. One of the things I dislike is the slow nature of such programs. Once oil is found, you are at the mercy of fluctuating oil prices for years to come as to what profit your investment returns. This aspect alone, having no control at all over a critical factor in this investment's success (the price of oil), violates all of my rules for investing today. However, it was not this limited partnership, but the second one I invested in where I received my real investment education.

I liked this second program's approach because management received no money until every investor got 125% of their initial investment returned. The drilling programs hit *big!* We projected (the company and I) about a 300% return! Now, recall the "limited partner" status for a moment.

The management of the program decided to combine all the different programs they had created in all the years their company had existed into one entity and issued shares of stock for their estimated value. I screamed. Class action law suits were filed. As limited partners we had no control over the operation of the company. We were completely at the "mercy" of the company's officers. The program officers were keeping a huge amount of the stock for themselves. The program owners (i.e., not the limited partners) made millions. I sold my shares of stock a year ago finally to take a tax loss (I kept hoping the stock would do better). My initial investment was $5,000. At one point the estimated worth of my share of the partnership exceeded $15,000! *My shares sold for $47.* I had quite a nice little tax loss to write off! (At least my accountant was pleased.)

This is a much shortened version of the story (the tears in my eyes make it difficult to write). What I learned was *not to give another person control over my financial future.* When the controlling partners decided to issue the stock, I could tell I was in real trouble, but other than yelling on the phone, there was nothing I could do. So for $5,000 I learned to not invest in ventures where I have no control. At least that is what I should have learned. Did I? Let's see.

LIMITED PARTNERSHIPS, TV

I know, it's still a limited partnership, but this was different! It was a local venture, and all the people involved were my friends, or at least acquaintances. All the investors were people for whom I had a great deal of respect. The investment offered an annual return of 20%! The idea was to go into small towns in our area and set up a cable TV system. We would have the only system available, because the city council would grant our company monopoly status in cable for their community before we invested. The man who had come up with the concept would run the business personally. The price per share was $15,000.

After the programs were begun, all the investors got a nice tax deduction. Two years went by in silence. Somebody (not me) finally got worried and checked on the programs. (Five separate programs, each in different towns, with separate investors in each, had been set up.) What he found got all of the investors together in the hospital for a meeting.

Why the hospital? It was very convenient, since all the investors were *doctors.* Our mutual accountant had brought us this investment opportunity. We were lucky in one respect. Since we had no lawyers or accountants among the investors, the hospital served as a great central location for all the M.D., dentist, and veterinarian investors to meet. The hospital was also convenient because the meetings involved considerable hemorrhage on the part of investors. But isn't that a strange coincidence: all the investors *happened* to be doctors? It's a quirk—a coincidence I still ponder.

I lost my $15,000. A dentist friend lost $45,000, almost all the savings he had. The guy who developed the concept and ran the program for us limited partners (much too busy as professionals to soil our hands in management) had just abandoned it. The fact that he personally went bankrupt was no solace to me. It took us about two months of meetings (at least I now more fully understand the expression "twisting in the wind") to realize we had lost everything. Great tax write-off, though. You can only write off $3,000 in losses per year. My dentist friend of the $45,000 investment has 15 years of deductions lined up. I bet his *new* accountant is just tickled by that fact!

An investment with a 20% yield projected? That is such a tremendous yield, it is close to violating the Iowa usury laws. No headaches either; someone else did all the work. I was a limited partner; just sit back and rake it in. I believe it was a good investment for me though. This time I think (hope and pray) that I really did learn my lesson.

If you have a "chance" to invest in a program that promises you a huge yield, ask yourself one question: if this is a good investment, why is the developer of the concept paying me so much more than it would cost him to borrow the money needed to fund the project from the bank? Let me save you the thought process. The answer is simple. The deal smells so badly no bank will let this guy in their building. He is forced to go to greedy and financially unsophisticated doctors to get money.

REAL ESTATE

Three of us set out in the early 1980s to make our fortune in the lucrative field of real estate. Many popular books had been written on making fortunes in this field. I think a general investment guideline is that when a book has been published and becomes popular in any given investment area, the opportunities for gain in that field are no longer extant.

I was to purchase the real estate (apartments were our area of "specialization"). A friend was to manage the properties for me and be paid a fee. Another friend was to oversee the physical condition of the buildings and make needed repairs. Of course, I'd pay him for the work he'd do. We all went together to select the investment properties. However, I went to the bank alone to sign the loan notes.

My friend who was to run the properties moved away a few months after we purchased two apartment buildings. Our maintenance expert wasn't very diligent in the performance of his obligations. We were forced to find other people to do this work. I replaced the manager—with my wife. I'm really glad she isn't writing this. I believe she would be forced to admit she did learn a lot in the years we managed the apartments. I also believe being set on fire would also prove "educational." It may even be more fun than running two apartments.

One good thing did occur due to my wife managing these properties. If I ever decide to look at real estate investing again, I'm sure my spouse will kill me. It's reassuring to know I can't make that mistake twice.

Boy, did we get tax breaks! We lost thousands. Our financial situation did get better after we locked the doors on one apartment building. The heating bills alone on that property were more than our total rent income in winter months, so closing it was an easy decision. Our losses were much less with the building empty. After we locked up the building, it was vandalized. We did have to go to court concerning that issue, but again, a learning experience. (One of the things we learned is that we didn't get any money over the vandalism issue. The judge awarded it to us, but the typical vandal is not noted for promptness towards financial obligations.)

I don't know how much we lost in total dollars. I never want to know. I do know how many calls we had because the toilet didn't work, usually due to a toy in it. (The renters didn't have to pay the plumber.) The day we sold the last apartment, just seven short and carefree years after we put it on the market, was a happy day for all of us! I felt *good*. I had bargained pretty cleverly, and on my wits alone I talked the purchaser into paying one-third of our original purchase price! We would have taken a lot less.

I learned enough in the world of real estate to write a whole second book. Let me sum up my advice in this fashion: If you want to buy real estate, why not give my wife a call first. Plan on a long conversation.

I have friends who have done well in real estate (or so they say). It's probably OK, if you have nothing else to do, are handy at fixing things, and have a keen sense of business. We got to meet some renters that were unlike any people I ever dreamed existed. The stay of one lady and her two children who were briefly our tenants proved so educational we actually paid them a month's rent to move out.

We could have had them thrown out for the things they had done. It would have taken a lawyer about three months to accomplish this task. Of course, by then it wouldn't have mattered. I doubt the building could have taken more than a month of the abuse they dished out before it committed suicide. Paying them to move, in retrospect, was a moment of brilliance on our part. Another learning experience!

These are all the losses I've managed to personally rack up in 20 years of investing. I have to date not lost a dollar in stocks, bonds, money market funds, or similar ventures. I guess that makes them pretty boring, huh?

I know of a lot of other pretty sure ways to "develop some tax write-offs." I have heard it said that no one ever makes money long term in the world of futures. Futures are contract to deliver a certain amount of goods, ranging from gold to hog bellies, at a set price on a set future date. The price you will buy the goods for is guaranteed. If the price of the commodity you have purchased goes up during the time period of the contract, you make money. If it goes down, you lose. These investments are leveraged: you control about 10 times the product you actually pay for. That means your gains are ten times as large as the change in the actual price of the commodity you invested in. So are your losses.

I know personally of no one who ever made a long-term profit playing commodities. I have several friends who have bought contracts in the futures market periodically, and one who wanted to make his living trading these financial instruments full time. All of them lost money and have quit this enterprise.

I once almost bought precious stones over the phone from a guy named Louie (no kidding). I have been approached to buy gold contracts, art, and a few other things that share this one common thread: *I knew nothing about them.* I want to assure you of one truth about these somewhat esoteric investment vehicles: Someone does make money on them. That person is the salesman.

I think I would be remiss if I didn't mention plain old-fashion gambling. This has been a growth industry of sorts in my native Iowa. The state backed a horse racetrack called "Prairie Meadows." They should have named it "Road Apples," I guess. It went broke, and the people who purchased the bonds issued to fund the track may have a problem.

We have also entered the world of riverboat gambling here in the heartland. One of the first legal gambling boats in Iowa, if not the United States of America, was based right in my home town of Keokuk, Iowa. The boat has recently left us to move on to the great state of Mississippi. Multiple law suits have been filed. Do any of you try lotto?

I can't begin to explain all of the permutations and variations of investments that have been developed. Most of them seem to have been born for the express purpose of allowing dentists to get rich quickly! My advice to you concerning all these schemes is that you don't need to study or understand them, if you understand the principles behind solid investing. Puts, calls, futures contracts, art, gems: lump them all under "things I don't need to understand, except to avoid." There is no such thing as get rich quick (except for the people who *sell* these programs).

You guard against these financial debacles by:

1. Knowing that many people exist in the financial community who have a great deal more information, training, and expertise in these areas than you will ever attain. If you allow them to persuade you in investment matters, you are at risk.

2. Don't invest your money where someone else controls the decision-making process.

3. *High return = High risk.* Tattoo this motto on your forehead! When someone talks to you of 100% returns, place your hand on your wallet. Don't let go.

4. Be aware of your limitations in the investment world. You have no training, no experience, and no time. Does this sound like the ideal preparation for someone entering into a complex investment situation?

5. In lieu of rule four, remember in matters financial to KISS. (Keep It Simple Stupid.) Awareness of ignorance contains its own reward.

Many people want the money you have earned as the fruits of your years of labor. It's *up to you* to see they don't get it. Clarify your values, and then set up an investment plan. Share this plan with your team. Don't try to get rich quick by investing in fly-by-night investment schemes. Stick with your plan instead. Try to work hard, be smart, and earn what you get. The great majority of doctors handle enough money in their lifetimes, to become wealthy through their professions if they deal with the money properly.

What's your life's goal as it pertains to money? Is it to impress the neighbors? Is it to find the easy way to do things? Is it *hoping* to one day be a success? Please don't laugh at these descriptions before you first examine your actions. What you see may surprise you. The greedy, those who want what they haven't earned (like a 20% return), are the ones who get taken. There is an old saying well worth reflecting on: "You can't cheat an honest man." I think this refers to a man determined to *earn* his rewards in life.

CONCLUSION

This has been a lot of fun to write. I hope you could sense that by what I've written. The purpose of my efforts is to share with you what I believe to be the potential that all in our profession possess. Every dentist has battled through an academic course that was extremely difficult to complete. It took great intelligence, but more than that, it took courage and tenacity to complete the years of study leading to the degree we obtained. I believe sometimes we forget to be proud of this singular accomplishment. Few in life have matched what we have achieved during our years of formal education, and yet we so often have taken this accomplishment for granted.

The job we do every day is, I believe, one of the most difficult in the world to perform. Restoring teeth would be demanding if you could hold the tooth in your hand while the procedures were being completed. (I may even be able to accomplish it then.) We have to do this task inside the mouth, in the dark and wet. Besides that, the mouth is attached to a wiggling, cowardly person who often won't hold still. These wiggly cowards also often won't pay their bills.

It is my firm belief that all of us who survived the basic training of eight years of college and can perform the difficult tasks of modern dentistry are capable of almost any accomplishment. By comparison, Rocky had it easy!

I wish I could tell you why our education system leaves us totally unprepared to run a dental *business*. Sad as our lack of formal preparation is, I know all of us have the potential to achieve financial success. We have to once again summon up our strength and make another great effort to learn, grow, and achieve, but we have been making these kinds of efforts most of our lives.

I hope my story illustrates that financial success and joy in dentistry are possible. All of what I've achieved has occurred in the Midwest during difficult economic times. Certainly being one of eight dentists in a town of 13,000 should show that my success wasn't based on any geographic fluke or finding the perfect location for a practice. I believe that the success I've documented in this book suggests what I have accomplished is *possible* for anyone who reads this and is willing to do what is necessary to obtain that which he/she desires.

The key, of course, is philosophy. Dare to do what so few will: sit quietly and learn to know your own heart. You must develop a focus that is true for you. No one can or should tell you what that focus may be. It could be wealth, fame, or the consistent display of love and joy to those about you. It may well be all three. The answer lies within you.

So know your heart, and from that wisdom, form a plan. Write that plan down, and reflect on it continually. Your plan will never be complete, because you will never cease to grow. Begin to examine your every thought and action by this premise: is this consistent with my goals? Attempt to adjust your behavior until the answer to this query is consistently *yes*.

Now that your plan is formed and becoming a part of your life, share it with your team. The team could be your staff, your family, or the Sunday school class you are a part of. Who makes up the team will be decided by the goals themselves. Continue to articulate your plan, and surround yourself with people who understand and believe in what you stand for. Nothing can stop talented people who truly believe in a worthy goal.

One last thing. No one fails. If you make a good effort, you produce results. These results should be reasons for joy. The goal you have set is really a beacon. The job of this beacon is to guide you on the right *path*. It is the journey, ever closer to your goal, that is the point. At least during life, we can never reach our goals; they constantly change and move ahead of us. Each day we are allowed to spend on this epic journey of life should fill us with joy.

If your life is filled with sorrow, you have strayed from *your* path. Stop, and study where you are. You have the power to correct yourself and resume the journey, no matter how far or for how long you have strayed. Let your feelings guide you, and continue to move toward joy.

If you feel I can somehow help you on your journey, call me at home. My number is 217–847–2816.

INDEX